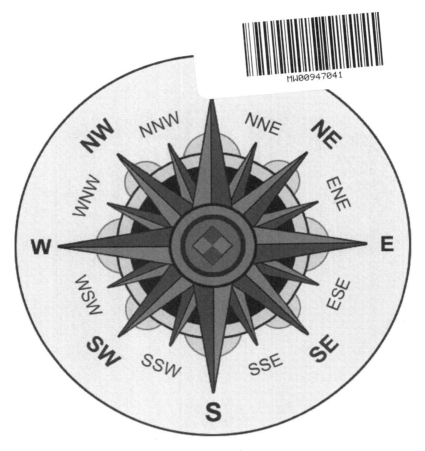

The Husband's

Field Guide

Navigating Your Wife's Essential Oil Habit

Andrew Edwin Jenkins

The Husband's Field Guide: Navigating Your Wife's Essential Oil Habit
by Andrew Edwin Jenkins

To learn more about The Field Guide,
please contact the author at:

www.TheHusbandsFieldGuide.com

www.Facebook.com/TheHusbandsFieldGuide
www.Facebook.com/AndrewEJenkins

www.Twitter.com/AndrewEJenkins

ISBN-10: 1497557666

ISBN-13: 978-1497557666

Library of Congress Control Number:

Cover Design: Robert Starnes
Photo Credits: Back cover & pages 244, 246, Natalie Spargo, Sez Me Photography

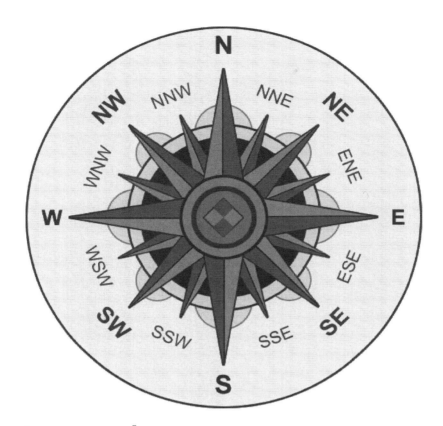

The Husband's

Field Guide

Navigating Your Wife's Essential Oil Habit

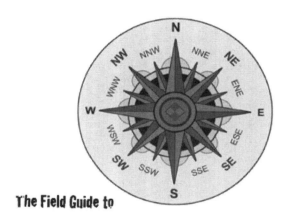

The Field Guide to

The Comp Plan

(A supplement to The Husbands' Field Guide: Navigating Your Wife's Essential Oil Habit)

Andrew Edwin Jenkins

www.TheHusbandsFieldGuide.com

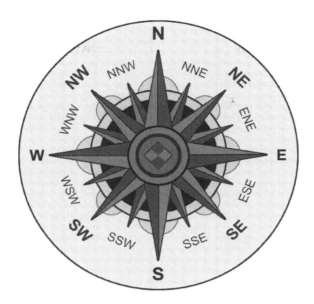

Dedication & thanks

Thanks to all the guys who had a part in the book- who shared their stories and taught me what they know. You guys have pushed me to walk in greater health and wholeness, and to do so with more compassion and humility. Thank you.

This book is dedicated to Cristy, my beautiful angel. I'm honored to travel this road with you. I am so proud of you- and so proud to be with you. You are an incredible mother, a fabulous wife, and an amazing everything-else-you-do. I ~~hope you are~~ know you will be far more successful with your business than you ever imagined possible!

I love you. So much.

Let's connect online

 www.Facebook.com/TheHusbandsFieldGuide
www.Facebook.com/AndrewEJenkins

 www.Twitter.com/AndrewEJenkins

 www.Vimeo.com/AndrewEJenkins

 www.TheHusbandsFieldGuide.com

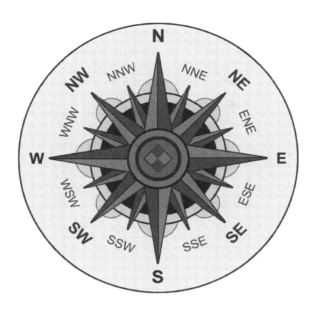

What others are saying about
The Field Guide

I love this book! Andy's field guide is chock full of valuable information, testimonies and engaging stories that will take you from the ultimate skeptic to the full blown oil fanatic!

Kelli Houck Wright, Young Living Distributor since October 2012
Diamond, Co-Founder of The Lemon Droppers
Birmingham, Alabama

Full of wit, humor and practical advice, Andy's field guide for husbands provides real world guidance for couples to realize success together despite hectic lives. A must read for husbands who want to discover what that smell is and why their wife is so excited about it, but don't know where to begin.

Scott Johnson, Young Living's Director of Global Education & U.S. Sales
Author of *TransformWise* & *Surviving When Modern Medicine Fails*

Almost every Young Living husband I've met has been there - your wife sits at the table, surrounded by a group of small bottles, asking you to smell them, telling you how incredible they are, and then suggesting she wants to try a home business. You stare back in disbelief, wondering if she was bitten by the snake that gave her the oils. Then, slowly, over time, you realize - she was right! The oils are amazing! They work! And, there is a real prospect with this company!

Well, Andy Jenkins, in his new Field Guide, helps minimize the time it will take you to go from a skeptic to a cheerleader to a willing partner in an incredible business venture! Sharing his personal story, and those of others, Andy writes a compelling and clear guide to help men see the oils through the leaves. This is a must read book for any man whose wife has started on the journey of taking control of her family's health and wellness, and who also has a desire for purpose and abundance.

James McDonald, Young Living Distributor since March 2010
Platinum
Morton, Illinois

Andy Jenkins has hit a HOME RUN! As a Christian, a husband, a father, and an entrepreneur, I found Andy's approach to explaining the Young Living opportunity not only very informative, but entertaining as well. His experiences & insights as a businessman & a family man will help anyone – (male or female) that wants to know what Young Living is really all about. This book is much more than just information though – I guarantee that it will change lives!

Mike Marlow, Young Living Distributor since June 2013
Executive
Kansas City, Missouri

The Husband's Field Guide not only gives practical advice for men to support their wive's YLEO business but also provides action steps to juggle many of life's high demands. The book is relatable... as each chapter gives a personal account from seven men who's wives have built large and successful organizations. Most importantly, after reading this book I have developed clear and concise action steps and goals to help our family run a successful business!!!

David Sheffield, Young Living Distributor since February 2013
Silver
Alabaster, Alabama

A great read that's entertaining, encouraging, equipping, and challenging all at once- A business building couple's must have.

Clint Ballard, Young Living Distributor since October 2012
Silver
Siloam Springs, Arkansas

The business side of Young Living has been typically a female dominated industry. It is so refreshing reading from the supportive husbands point of view! There are more and more men jumping on board. Can't wait to share this book with many! Thanks, Andy, for your time and effort in this book!

Heidi Ross, Young Living Distributor since August 2012
Platinum
Red Deer, Alberta, Canada

I know you, man. You're a skeptic just like me. Your wife is getting into all this "live natural" stuff, and now she wants to spend 100 bucks on a little bottle of oil that wouldn't even fill a shot glass! Well, if you want to understand why, read Andy's story here. It's my story, too, and the story of many guys who have come to realize their wives were right about Young Living essential oils. Read it, take it to heart. The information in this book will change your life.

Gary Edwards, Young Living Distributor since 2010
Gold
Fort Frances, Ontario, Canada

Andy gives practical advice for men ready to leave the sidelines and partner with their wife as they grow a thriving business. It has been incredibly rewarding to minister together, to friends and loved ones, through sharing Young Living Essential Oils! Interacting with other couples like Andrew and Cristy has my wife and I even more excited to pursue this venture together.

Spencer Thornburg, Young Living Distributor since July 2013
Gold
San Diego, California

As a husband of an 'oiler' sometimes it is hard to know what to do or how to do it for your wife in order to help her achieve her goals in her business. This is a challenge to say the least- even if you are willing. Every man wants / needs a challenge in his life, something to give his life purpose, as well as direction. The Husband's Field Guide does just that. It provides a challenge to do and to be more for her and gives simple instructions on how to get there.

Michael Wight, Young Living Distributor since January 2013
Platinum
Calera, Alabama

Definitely an "Out of the Oilers Closet" experience!!! Andy has aced it, straight to the point in the experience as a male essential oil user. This is it!!!

Juan Alberto Arevalo, Young Living Distributor since July 2013
Executive
Culiacan, Sinaloa, Mexico

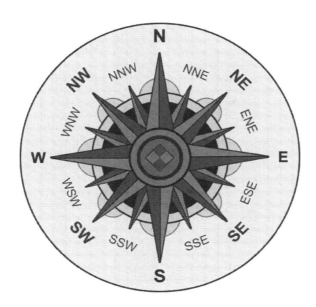

Table of contents

Foreword   i

Intro: the next best step   1

01: You can't make this stuff up   15

01: Direction: get started   33

01: Take these meds forever, or… / Marty's story   35

02: The trees are for the healing of the nations   41

02: Direction: re-read your history   65

02: A diffuser is a what? / Verick's story   67

03: Essential oils 101   71

03: Direction: learn a little   105

03: Out of my comfort zone / Stephen's story   109

04: How I got here   113

04: Direction: get comfortable with it   149

04: Try something new / Les's story   153

05: Getting traction   157

05: Direction: know how it works   173

05: It almost seems unfair… / Josh's story   177

06: Reverse engineer your life   181

06: Direction: work it   199

06: Together / Kent's story   201

07: Raise the water level   205

07: Direction: get a little bit better every day 229

07: The rest is history / Jeremiah's story   233

Final thought: keep enjoying the next best step 237

Resources for further study   241

About the author   245

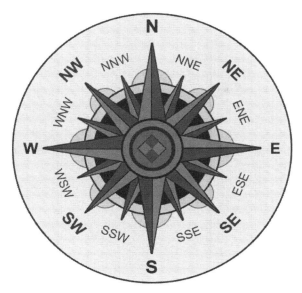

Foreword

Dave Braun & Troy Amdahl / @OolaSeeker & @OolaGuru

We are passionate everything Oola. We write about it, speak about it, coach about it, and post about it to anyone who will listen. What is Oola? Oola is a life that is balanced and growing in all key areas of health and well-being. It is a state of awesomeness in which your life is balanced and growing in the seven areas of life as you move towards experiencing the life you dream of and deserve. We call the key areas the 7 F's of Oola (Fitness, Finance, Family, Field, Faith, Friends, and Fun).

As we teach about Oola, "balance" seems to attract much of the attention. In this fast paced world with endless demand for our time, a more balanced life is often the goal. If you're a guy and find yourself wading through this "new craze" of essential oils, you may feel like a few things are out of balance. You probably already thought you were busy, and now your wife has added *another* thing to your family's "to do" list. You may feel like 7 is a lot of F's. You'd probably settle for 2 or 3 on most days.

With all this focus on "balance", however, it's easy to forget the "grow" aspect. Each day it is important to make small steps toward being better and doing better in each of the 7 key areas of life. We encourage you to stop, take a look around, and see if your wife's new found hobby is, in fact, part of an OolaPath to your OolaLife. Perhaps she's found a vehicle that will help bring harmony to your Family, your Fitness, your Friends, your Field, your Faith… your Fun… and, yes, even your Finances. Is it possible her new passion is an opportunity for you and your family to "grow" *and* realize more "balance" at the same time?

The Husband's Field Guide assumes you know little to nothing about essential oils and / or running a multilevel home-based business. This books shows you step by step how to set and reach your business goals, while simultaneously building a better life. Written by a guy who self-admittedly knew nothing about the business or the oils, Andy Jenkins delivers a neat, tidy package that equips you in an easy-to-read format.

He'll give you action steps and questions to really think about. Some of these steps are glamorous, others seem mundane, but they are all steps in the right direction. You'll find these steps quickly put you on the road to your own OolaPath.

Oola is all about people doing better and being better. Both. Because Oola affects us internally and it changes things externally, we believe when you integrate the steps outlined in this book, and make them part of your daily routine, the first thing to change will be you. In turn, you'll help others, who will then help others…

Our entire mission is to help people realize their purpose and live an OolaLife. *The Husband's Field Guide* will help you do just that.

Visualize the life you want. Read Andy's book. See if it helps you get there. An OolaLife is worth the pursuit. You and your dreams are worth it.

#LiveOola and #ShareOola,

Dave Braun & Troy Amdahl

@OolaSeeker & @OolaGuru

Authors of the International Best Seller, *Oola: Find Balance in an Unbalanced World*

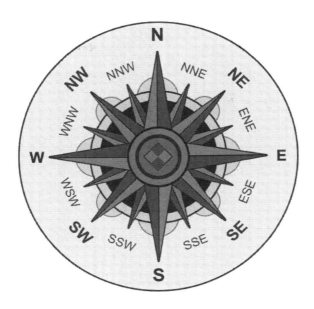

Intro: the next best step

I've got nine kids, a full-time job, and a bunch of other stuff going on. I preach about 3 times a month at a church in Birmingham.[1] On top of that, the nonprofit I run is opening a thrift store in the next 30 days.[2] That means long hours, lots of business decisions, overseeing the process, running construction plans, and leading my team. The store will be open by the

> **Main idea:** I want to make your wife's business important to you.

time you read this, meaning the whirlwind of life will have gotten even faster. To give you a taste of what my job at the nonprofit entails:

- We've had three company vehicles stolen- *at least*.[3] One of them was stolen two weeks after we received it, brand new, through a grant.

- I've been in more drug houses than most drug dealers.

---

[1] The Grace Church: www.GraceBirmingham.com

[2] The Village Thrift: www.TheVillageThrift.net. I'll write more about this later in the book.

[3] You know it's crazy when you can't even keep count of stuff like this!

- I've gone and retrieved stolen items, including those cars, directly from the people who stole them. And, yes, they had guns and I didn't.

- I've been physically threatened by pimps when they've called us looking for "their" girls. And I've assured them they'd have to go physically through me and my staff to get "their" girls back!

You see, just over six years ago we started a nonprofit that helps men, women, and families coming out of prison, off the streets, from jails, homelessness, and human trafficking. In the early days we actually housed some of these people in very close proximity to our home.

The first five male prisoners, each of whom came to us on early release, meaning they were still under the custody of the State of Alabama Department of Corrections, lived directly across the street from us in a rental house we own. The next crew lived down the street. Then we opened a house a block over. And a few apartments behind our house. Then an entire apartment complex down the street. Eventually there were 17 properties going. (We may or may *not* have had support from our neighborhood association.)

At one time we even had 6 women living in *our* home as the women's program was being born. One of our most valuable staff members, Jonette, who has overseen the women's program, served as the Director of Operations for the ministry, and is now helping run production at the new thrift store, was one of those women.

After about five weeks, the ladies moved out of our house when the ministry finally had a home ready for them. Not long after they moved out, we were blessed to partner with another amazing ministry called The Well House, led by founder and executive director, Tajuan McCarty. At that point we opened our home to the first The Well House rescued victims. We had an intermittent flow of women coming and going over the next month.

The thrust of our ministry and purpose has been simple: *change lives.*

Most people come to us with nothing more than a backpack, a suit case of belongings, or even just a brown paper grocery back with their name on it. That represents everything they have in the world. The majority have burnt the last few bridges they had and are eager to move forward. If they complete the six-to-nine-month residential recovery program, they will graduate with a full-time job, their court and legal issues will be resolved, and they will receive assistance relocating to a house or apartment of their own. They'll be drug free, have a ton of practical life skills, and they'll know the loving heart of their Heavenly Father.[4]

When we started doing this, there were no books written about how to do it, and none of it was popular. So we learned it all on the fly, picking up pieces of wisdom from others who were doing the same things and applying whatever lessons we learned the hard way.

The name of the ministry is The Village.[5] I named it that because I feel like, too often, Christians want to live in co-existence with one another, but not necessarily engaging in relationships that would spur us on toward love and good deeds. A village is a city within a city; a place where everyone pools their time, talents, and gifts together for the benefit of the whole. We started this ministry to encourage people not to push off the promises of God until the future- until we get to Heaven. It's my belief that healing and wholeness are possible now, regardless of the sickness. In other words, **Jesus didn't just come to take people to Heaven, He came to bring the presence of the Kingdom here.** *Now*.

I also feel that, often, the Church pulls away from people in the world- as if the world will taint us and make us "unclean." It's odd, because Jesus never lived that way. He *touched* lepers and adulterers and

> Jesus didn't just come to take people to Heaven, He came to bring the presence of the Kingdom here.

those in need, knowing that they wouldn't make Him unclean but that He would totally transform them and make them *completely* new.

The prophet Jeremiah, in the Old Testament, even told the Israelites who were in exile in Babylon (probably one of the most pagan, idolatrous cultures to date) and waiting for God to take them home that they should *not* look to escape from the world in which they were living, but to *serve* and *love* the people around them:

> *Build houses and live in them; plant gardens and eat their produce.*
> *Take wives and have sons and daughters; take wives for your sons, and*
> *give your daughters in marriage, that they may bear sons and*
> *daughters; multiply there, and do not decrease. But seek the welfare of*

---

[4] Here's a link to a video on our website with me explaining all of this in about 6 minutes: http://welcometothevillage.wordpress.com/who-we-are/

[5] www.WelcomeToTheVillage.net

the city where I have sent you into exile, and pray to the Lord on its behalf, for in its welfare you will find your welfare.[6]

Notice, Jeremiah tells them to plan to live long term in Babylon- and to do long terms things. Plant gardens, cultivate a family, and grow…

Jeremiah said to *love* and *serve* that city of man, even while living in the City of God. It's almost like you occupy two places at once. And that's the kind of life that Jesus modeled- one that lived the presence of The Kingdom while walking on the streets of another.

Anyway, back to my story…

Did I mention I'm trying to lose weight? As if all the responsibilities I've previously mentioned haven't caused your head to spin, I decided I should also drop a few pounds. I saw some pictures of myself a few weeks ago and realized I was no longer the lean, athletic version of myself that I used to be. Somehow, over the past decade, I've gradually moved into a state of physicality I'll call "festively plump." I don't even think that's a legit phrase, but *I'm owning it.*

I asked my wife about it. She sweetly told me I could stand to lose a little bit of weight. I could tell she didn't really want to be direct about it, because she didn't want to crush my pride. So, that's how she phrased it: I could *stand to…*

"Like how much?" I asked. Then, I tried to quantify it before she could answer: "Maybe 20 pounds?"

She looked at me and smiled. She motioned that I should go to a higher number.

"25?" I asked, slightly elevating the pitch of my voice, to accentuate the *five* and the finality of the number.

She motioned a bit higher…

"30?"

"Yeah, probably so," she told me. "You could do at least twenty five…" (*At least?* I thought.) "…but probably closer to 30 would do it."

Thirty pounds. There it was. The reality. And now, the goal.

Somehow, in the busy-ness of life, I let myself go. So I decided to get my physical self back into shape. I just happened to decide to do it while juggling my

---

[6] Jeremiah 29:5-7, English Standard Version.

plethora of responsibilities / jobs, raising nine kids, and doing a home-based network marketing business. Brilliant, I know.

I don't have time for one more thing. You probably don't either. **If I'm adding anything to my schedule, it has to be important. And beneficial. It has to make sense**.

Some weeks, I look across the bed and ask my wife, who may be typing a message to someone on our team or someone who wants info about essential oils, how it's *already* Thursday. "The week is gone," I tell her. "Didn't it just start?"

You know the routine; the time flies. They say it flies when you're having fun. I've noticed it pretty much flies whether you're having fun or not. And when you're busy chasing your tail most of the week. My days are feeling longer and longer, but the weeks seem shorter and shorter. Can you relate?

So why am I telling you all of this? Well, I wanted you to see a real, raw picture of my life before I launch into the nuts and bolts of this Field Guide.

Enter: Young Living. Just over eight months ago Cristy bought the Premium Starter Kit. I'll tell you that story later in the book. She honestly didn't have time to go out the night she met some friends to learn about the oils, which is probably why she *needed* to go. We're that busy.

But let me introduce you to my wife. She's incredibly talented. She manages our household, home schools the kids, and leads worship with the team at our church. She's a childbirth educator and a certified doula, meaning that she assists in

> *I don't have time for one more thing.* You probably don't either. If I'm adding anything to my schedule, it has to be important. And beneficial.

natural childbirth. She also serves as a doula liaison to one of the largest hospitals in our city. She also co-owns, helps manage, and leads Gentle Childbirth Services, LLC.

She is *amazing*. Absolutely amazing.

Eight weeks after she birthed our newest baby boy, Salter, she was invited to a meeting where Young Living essential oils were discussed and taught. Needing a well deserved break out of the house, she loaded the baby and off she went. She returned a Young Living believer!

Then, she started holding meetings and teaching about the oils, something she never planned to do (probably like you- I've been astounded at the number of people who get into Young Living simply to use the products and end up selling them), and our schedule got even tighter.

Sorry, I don't have time or energy for this

Over a year ago, The Village acquired a larger facility where we could move everyone- men on one wing of the facility, women on another, and families on another (our nonprofit is the first in town where married couples do not have to separate from each other or their children to receive overnight transitional housing services). We started an intern program to train future leaders, as well as relieve some of the pressure that was on our staff. Today we can house up to 150 people. Many of them have court and legal issues; most of them have relational things they are working through; some of them still struggle with addictions. Most of them are wonderful people, but the work is not easy or glamorous.

I naively thought that things would get *easier* when it got bigger. Parts of it did, and parts of it didn't. Not having to do everything myself (in the early days, I did most things, and have literally done *every* single job for a short season that we currently have at the ministry) has been easy. But budgets have gotten bigger (and more stressful) and the needs are vast. And there are more moving parts to our little ministry machine than there were in the early days.

Of course, as the numbers of people that are being served grow, the "5%" who choose to be trouble-makers grow too. The "squeaky wheels" people. Most of the people who come to us are incredibly grateful for a second chance at life, but 5 out of 100 clearly aren't. They'd rather cause trouble for us and everyone else. And that adds stress to everyone.

Somehow, when Cristy decided to work the business side of Young Living, I lumped it into that 5%. I know, it sounds odd. Young Living is not even part of my "day job" and I'd already equated a few of the things associated with her new hobby to the *worst* parts of my actual job:

- Week nights when the wife is away and I'm running the house on my own, getting the kids all fed, bathed, and into bed. (Have I mentioned she can do all that stuff blind-folded?)

- Trying to go to bed, because I've got a busy day ahead of me, but being unable to sleep because my wife has her computer on in the bed next to me- speakers blaring (she wants me to add here that she really didn't have the sound *that* loud) while someone explains the compensation plan *and* the clicking of the keyboard while she answers a few questions for clients or potential clients grating all at once.

- Coming home to a house that looks like a tidy is overdue, watching the kids zoom in and out of the back door, while the baby fusses for more Cheerios in the high chair- only to do some investigative work and find my wife talking quietly on the phone in our bedroom, behind a closed door (to block out the noise and chaos of her day to day world for just a moment), all because someone was having trouble "setting up their ER" or "trying to sign-up on their computer."[7]

Perhaps, you've probably "been there / done that" by now?

Because of this and my out-of-whack priorities (which I justified with my hectic schedule), I didn't help Cristy do her Young Living business at all. A few months ago, it was *her* business, her thing. **Now, although the business still *hers*, I feel more and more like it's *ours*.**

Until recently, my only historical involvement with the business consisted of wearing a t-shirt to an event in our hometown of Birmingham, Alabama. Young Living was unveiling the Ningxia Nitro at a

> Now, although the business is still *hers*, I feel more and more like it's *ours*.

local hotel and convention center. Our team, the Lemon Droppers, had a brilliant idea: *Let's create a t-shirt and all wear it to rally together and show our team spirit!*

Cristy asked me about attending the event: "Sure, I'll go with you."

She assured me other women were bringing their husbands, that I wouldn't be the only guy there.

Then a few days later she hit me with the t-shirt idea: "I'll wear it…" I *promised*.

Of course, other guys were sure to be wearing theirs, too. "Several wives are ordering them for their husbands," she explained to me. "They'll have theirs on, too."

We went to eat dinner with two of our friends before the event, Josh and Fredia. You'll meet Josh later in the book. He's a gifted tech kind of guy that can edit any kind of video and make any kind of musician sound like a professional. The first

---

[7] I'll explain these terms later.

thing I noticed about Josh was this: *no t-shirt*. He was dressed like he was going out to eat at a nice restaurant (which is exactly where we were meeting before heading to the Young Living event).

"No t-shirt?" I asked him.

He shrugged his shoulders and gave me a silent "*Nahhhhh*."

I looked to Cristy.

"There'll be other guys there… they'll have *their* shirts on," she reminded me.

Now, in fairness to her, she gave me a few "outs." And she is amazing (as I've told you), so she didn't have to sell me hard on the shirt idea.

As we approached the restaurant early in the evening, she told me I could put on a real shirt. I thought about Josh being the only guy with a t-shirt, then thought about what it would mean to her for me to wear the shirt… I told her I was persisting. After all, she'd been to plenty of my events- and she would have worn the t-shirt any of those times if we ever had them.

She gave me another out after dinner, after Josh showed up *sans* t-shirt. Then in the car on the way to the event. Then as we approached the building and I dropped her off at the door.

I remember peering through the window as I dropped her near the side entrance. Very few t-shirts. *Very few men.* I wore the shirt and, of course, I survived. I didn't cover it up with a jacket and no one made fun of me. At least to my face.

And when I look back at it, it's embarrassing to me that *that* t-shirt is the *only* support I had given her to this point in her entire business venture.

A little bit at a time = a whole bunch of progress

We have purposely chosen to embrace the opportunity that Young Living presents and treat this in the way that I've learned to treat the best parts of my job. I absolutely hate watching people fail drug tests and go back to prison. I detest it when someone chooses to take their check from their job on payday and go back to the crack house. It unsettles me when the ladies go back to a guy that's no good for them and is more interested in making a buck off them than tenderly loving them. But it all happens some of the time.

I love it when families are reunited. When people move into their own homes. When women come out of prostitution for good. When guys marry the "baby's momma."

None of that happens overnight, though. It takes time. So we operate off a concept that I articulate like this: **Incremental change over time is exponential.** That means this: a bunch of little changes- or a series of small steps- equals big change. Or, to say it another way, "If you do a bunch of small things consistently, the pay-off is huge."

When people come to us for help at The Village, we *know* that we can't reset their entire life in a single day. Some of them don't even have a past "good point" to reset to. We know that we must make a series of small changes… and then everything is transformed.

That's how we even try to run the organization. There are major projects we would love to do (and big ones that we've already done). I'm learning that time and patience and persistence will get you just about anywhere. Again, **a bunch of small changes are easier, more lasting, and often more significant than one big change when all are added together.**

You see this concept in action everyday…

> …a bunch of small changes are easier, more lasting, and often more significant than one big change when all are added together.

For example: The couch potato to five-K running plan acknowledges that most of us can't "cold turkey" go pound out 3.2 miles. But, with a bit of incremental change we can. It's exponential.

And, of course, though most of us are overwhelmed at the idea of plowing through the Bible quickly- as we do with self-help books and best-sellers- you can incrementally work through the entire thing. You can hit it in 90 days- or even run through the Bible in a year. Pick a plan. Again, incremental change is powerful.

You've seen how kids grow. You don't notice yours changing at all, day by day. Then, they go to the grandparents for a few days- and come back looking three years older. Again, small changes, though unnoticeable in the moment, add together making a large change.

I say that to say this: We often look at the progress that other people have made and we begin comparing their lives to our own. The problem (one of the many problems) with this is that **we most often compare the "greatest hits" / highlight reel of their life (what we see) to our ongoing struggle of the incremental minutia.** Yet everyone has the small baby steps they must deal with- we just don't see them.

Here's my encouragement to you about *any* area of your life:

- Determine what it is you want to do (write a novel, read a book, run a certain distance…)

- Break it into small steps (10 pages a day, some running plan, etc…)

- Don't be overwhelmed by the smallness of what you are achieving each day.

- Keep achieving it- take that small step each day. *Then,*

- Step back and look at the change… one week later… one month… three months…

Right now, I'm doing this with weight loss. I decided to lose the 30 pounds. I started that *the very same day* I started writing this book. I literally opened up a new Pages document in my MacBook Air for the draft of this book and a Numbers spreadsheet for the weight loss regimen. (That was the day that we were leaving Hawaii, the trip I'll tell you about later which we took that *totally* changed my outlook on Young Living.) I set some step-by-step goals. I started tracking my journey and watching my progress towards accomplishing those goals.

I'm finally living out an example of what I thought to be true all along. In health & fitness, incremental changes- a bunch of small steps strung together- have a huge impact.

The same is true in your Young Living business. Small steps. Lots of them. Some of them so small that you'll wonder if you're actually making any progress at all. One enrollment at a time. One bit of new knowledge at a time. One class at a time. One more step…

You will see your influence grow. Small at first. And then more.

You will watch your bank accounts change. A bit at a time. Then faster.

You will watch your organization's size blossom. A few at a time. Then a dozen at a time. Then *hundreds* at a time.

Nuts & bolts

There are seven "real" chapters in this book and an appendix. I'm going to walk you through the following train of thought:

- My first exposure to Gary and Young Living (Chapter 1: You can't make this stuff up)

- What I've learned about essential oils and their use throughout history, including the Bible times (Chapter 2: The trees are for the healing of the nations)

- The basic facts of essential oils- what they are and how we get them (Chapter 3: Essential oils 101)[8]

- My involvement with my wife's business, as well as how I got comfortable with network marketing (Chapter 4: How I got here)

- Steps that will help you move forward in the business if you choose to do so (Chapter 5: Getting traction)

- I've also included some steps to take to reorient your life and build towards a more preferred future that involves your business as well as the rest of your life (Chapter 6: Reverse engineer your life, Chapter 7: Raise the water level)

After each of these chapters, I've included two more smaller chapters. One is titled "Direction" and the other is always "Somebody's story." So twenty-one things to read in all- then a final thought and the appendix.

...let's start walking. We've got a few next best steps to take.

The "Direction" chapters will provide you with some *easy* next steps. I give you articles to read, specific chapters of books to review (so you don't have to read the entire thing), videos to go watch online, and even a few tasks to do. Some of these activities will work great for you- some of them may not. If it helps you put

---

[8] Think of this as a Clif Notes version of a non-existent "Essential oils for dummies" book.

things together, do it; if it doesn't, scrap it. If you find something better, email it to me and I'll put it in the next edit of the book and cite your name as my source. I really think we can do better together than we each do alone. So, let's figure it out.

The "Somebody's story" chapters are probably ~~some of~~ the best in the book. We've met some incredible men and women through Young Living. I called some of the guys in our upline (meaning they are way ahead of us in the process of building their business), and several in our downline (meaning they're not quite where we are). That will give you a variety of perspectives. I asked them to share their stories and how they got involved with Young Living. You'll find that, for the most part, their wives were onboard well before they were. Just like mine.

Their stories are honest, transparent, and something you'll probably easily relate to. You'll learn a great deal from them.

Tonight, I called my friend Stephen, a youth minister I've known since high school, and asked him to write one of these chapters. He, according to some of the women who were at the Essential Oils 101 class that his wife hosted in their home, light heartedly joked about "snake oils" and "voodoo".

"I was what they call a late adopter," he confessed as we spoke about this book.

We couldn't help but laugh.

He then told me something we can all agree on, **"It seems like there aren't a lot of easy places for *guys* to go get information about the oils**." Some brilliant women in our upline created a large FaceBook group where people can post questions and testimonials. The Lounge, as we call it, contains a lot of great info. But some of it is more "mom-specific." Things like what to do with a kid that has a snotty nose. The Lounge answer: get out *X*, *Y*, and *Z* oils. The usual guy answer: *blow the nose*.

I told Stephen that I hope this book will be a great resource for guys- at least a simple place to hit the ground running. I think in reading stories like his and some of the other guys' testimonials- a state trooper, a guy who works in an ER, an audio-visual tech… I think you'll learn some things you can use, too.

Plus, if you're like me, you'll probably hear it better from other guys than from your wife. I don't know *why* it is that guys do that, but we do. I read stuff on the Internet, or hear it from one of my guy friends and then tell Cristy, "Guess what I just learned?!" I'll excitedly fill her in on the latest and greatest, only to be reminded (rightly) that she informed me about _____ *months* ago.

Sometimes, she humors me by saying, *"Really?" How interesting,"* with a sly smile and raised eyebrow.

If you're like me, you'll probably experience the same thing with your wife as you read through these pages and tell her some great thing that you're hearing for the "first" time. Odds are, she's already told you. I guarantee you that she knows more about essential oils than me- and probably more than the guys I'll introduce over the next few pages.

How the book works

Part of the book	What it is / does
Chapters 1-7	Provides you with information
Direction	Gives you some practical tools, research, or next steps to take- there is one of these after each of the chapters
Somebody's story	Shows you how someone else is applying this stuff in their own life- there is one of these, too, after each chapter

Yes, I have an agenda

Ah… one more thing. Yes, I have an agenda here. I know as a guy I'm always thinking, *What's this person's angle? What do the really want?*

Here it is: **I want to make your wife's business important to you.** If you grabbed this book on your own, it probably already is. If she picked it up and passed it to you, there it is… now you know my angle.

Cristy and I were walking near the lava-covered beaches in Hawaii. I'd already told her that I was going to help her with her business when we got back home. Again, until that point, I'd only worn the shirt. Once. And you know how I felt about that.

"What are you going to *do*?" she asked. "What way do you think you can help the most...?"

I told her, "I think the thing that I'm best at is making things simple. I'm hoping I can figure out a way to communicate this stuff in an easy to understand way..."

> **I'm not selling you *anything*...**
> You've *already* paid in. Whether or not you receive all of the benefits of this is now up to you.

Then I added, "I think we've got to make it important to the guys / husbands. If we make it important to the guy, the business will soar higher."

"I don't think you can do *that*?" she said, somehow making the statement a question. "You can't make something important to someone else, can you?"

I told her that I thought she was half-way right. I *can't* make something important to you. But I can show you the tremendous opportunity that sits within your reach. Hopefully, you'll find that to be true in this book- that we'll take some complex things and make them ultra-easy to understand. That's part of the aim, anyway.

Let's face it. **I'm not selling you *anything*.** You're wife has probably already bought into the essential oil madness (I say that in the most endearing way possible), meaning you already have a starter kit, complete with a diffuser and a pile of oils that you- if you're like me- don't know what exactly to do with. You've *already* paid in. Whether or not you receive all of the benefits of this is now up to you.

That said, let's start walking. We've got a few next best steps to take.

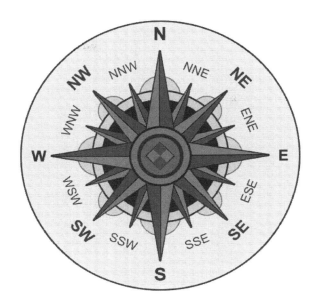

01: You can't make this stuff up

I heard a lot about Gary Young before I met him.

At the Ningxia Nitro event in Birmingham, Alabama, Jared Turner, one of the executives at Young Living, took the stage and talked about the culture of the company I've come to admire and love so much.[9] You probably have, too, or you wouldn't be reading this book.

Somewhere in the midst of his PowerPoint facts and figures about sales and growth trends, Jared scrolled to a pic of Gary snapped from behind. Gary probably had no

> **Main idea:** Some things that seem too good to be true are actually good and true.

idea he was getting photographed. In fact, as the story goes, he made *everyone* at the dinner party late for dinner.

---

[9] http://www.youngliving.com/en_US/products/wellness/liquid-wellness/ningxia-nitro

Gary sat on a stool in front of a distiller- a large metal drum that looks like an over-sized keg. He was wearing a long-sleeve outdoor-type button down shirt and his hat.

"This is what it's all about," Jared told the crowd. "We were all waiting to eat… time came to say grace, we all scanned the room, and Gary was nowhere to be found…"

He relayed how they looked a few places for him, but then apparently had no doubt as to where he might be.

"We walked to the distiller… it was the first time Ponderosa Pine was coming out of the machines… and there was Gary, late at night… sitting in the dark… just waiting to check the final product."

As an attorney-turned-world-traveler with the rest of the Young Living crew, Jared relayed an even greater appreciation for a man whose primary role would, you'd think, have him behind a desk somewhere in a penthouse office. Apparently, **Gary had graciously bucked all of those rules without even knowing such rules exist somewhere in the corporate world.** He is a CEO that checks his own distillers and, as I'd later come to learn, takes dangerous treks to places in the world where others probably wouldn't go.

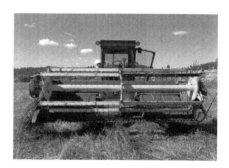

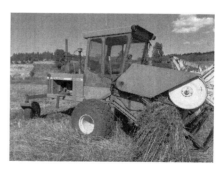

Craig Aramaki, who was leading the marketing efforts for Young Living at the time, told a quick story about one of his visits to Gary.[10] I'm not sure if it was an interview, or a check-in for progress, or what…

---

[10] Craig Aramaki was the Chief Marketing Officer from February 2013 to February 2014. He has since left the corporate side of YL to work as an independent distributor. See his extremely gracious post explaining this move on his February 16, 2014 FaceBook status. It shows you the enormous opportunity that is in the field, that an executive level staff member left the office to go work as a distributor.

Gary was in the field driving a "swather." It'a large tractor-looking thing, like a small combine. It was time to harvest one of the plants for distilling, Tansy.

The way Craig tells the story, with his infectious smile and bright eyes, Gary jumped out of the tractor, left the engine running, and then coaxed Craig behind the wheel. A few minutes later, Craig was driving…

Not long after that, Gary was off to the next task… more harvesting, more distilling…

Craig worked the tractor *all day*. That's right. All. Day. Long.

"You can't match his work ethic," Craig said. "And to see a CEO that could sit back and relax, take a break…but is still the first one in the field and the last one out… *amazing.*"

Yes, he was going for a meeting and wound up working the field. A day of pencil-pushing turned into a day of moving mud and earth. That's just how it goes. By the way, those are Craig's pictures of the actual swather.

I don't know of any stories of Gary that exist from his high school or college years. I'm sure they're there, but I got the impression that he was the kind of true-to-life legend that you hear about… the "greatest hits" version of all the other cool kids all wrapped into one.

There were so many stories of people's oddly fun interactions with Gary, that parts of the Birmingham event sounded more like a "Gary and Mary" introduction than a Ningxia Nitro event. It was clear that the people all *adored* this man.

> I got the impression that he was the kind of true-to-life legend that you hear about… the "greatest hits" version of all the other cool kids all wrapped into one…

The haters can hate

Of course, not everyone loves him. Some people actually dislike him very much- and go to all lengths possible to let others know. We have friends- even close friends- who have completely ignored the benefits of Young Living and what the oils can do for them because of the trash they've read on the Internet.

For instance, one lady called us one day- *persistently*. She called once. Then twice. Then again. Each time she left a similar message: She wanted us to drop what we were doing (with nine kids!) so that she could come get some of the oils. She said it in a really nice way, of course. I think she thought we had a small stock of inventory from which we sold the oils (some people do; we didn't at the time). And I think she thought our store (which we don't have) was always open for business.

When she got my wife on the line she told Cristy something like this: "I saw your video online," she said, referring to the training video Cristy created (I'll tell you more about that later, too).[11] "I really believe God sent me to these oils," she continued, "because I've been praying about healing for some very specific things in my family…"

This kind and gracious lady we know through several mutual friends continued calling about the oils. She wanted several. And she wanted them *right then*. We would have given them to her, but we didn't stock kits at the time and, even if we did, we weren't at home and were running around for a full day of activities. With nine kids, it seems like we're always delivering, picking up, dropping off, getting, chasing or recalculating something in our daily schedule- even though most of what we do we actually do together.

When Cristy was able to finally get to her she said something like this: "Well… I don't know, now…"

Then we got the scoop. She found the World Wide Web blogosphere land mines.

"I looked up some things on the Internet about Gary Young and I'm not sure…"

I looked at Cristy and told her, "Well, I'm glad we didn't change our whole schedule to get that to her… Maybe God didn't tell her so clearly. Or maybe she exercised a little veto…"

Cristy and I laughed, shrugged the whole thing off, and moved to the next item on the "to do" list.

I want to show you the persuasive power of the Internet, for good and bad.

---

[11] Short version: Cristy created an online class that she doesn't have to be at when it happens. She recorded herself teaching about the oils, so that she can send it to her team to use if they don't feel comfortable teaching the information. As well, instead of teaching the class in "real time" (like a webinar), people can log on at any time with the password. We found that some people are reluctant to go to an introductory class at someone's home (or even a restaurant). Many times that's just because they're already overextended and busy. They don't have a free night to give to get somewhere at a specific time- but they can sit at their laptop after they put the kids to bed.

- The speed and ease with which you can handle Young Living orders and run your business: *good*.

- The uses for essential oils you'll be able to find through podcasts and other links: *good*.

- You might have picked up this book from the Internet: *that's good!*

- The ungracious chatter that's out there: *definitely bad.*

> Didn't Jesus say you would know them by their fruit? Not by their excessive words or self-proclaimed greatest hits version of themselves?

The Internet itself is not bad, but it certainly provides the opportunity for so-called "haters" to express themselves. And, unfortunately, haters seem to bog it down. They're like the 5% of guys that cause trouble for us in our nonprofit. These bloggers have about 2% of the total bandwidth that's out there, but they make it buzz like it's 98%- and they make it sound like no one has anything positive to say at all.

And, look, I'm probably not bringing up anything you haven't already looked at. When my wife got into Young Living, I googled the company out of curiosity and read *most* of what I found. I decided this:

- The people who are writing venom aren't writing to simply caution you about oils; they're writing to digitally body slam and functionally discredit Gary. In other words, **they have an agenda that's not simply informational in nature, it's personal and- dare I say it- dysfunctional**. And since when is the Internet really the best place to air out a personal or relational difference with someone?

- **The oils work.** Therefore, I eliminated all of their rebuttals that were "scientific" or "research-proven." Most are just long-winded arguments that killed a lot of trees to write or occupied extra megabytes in the blogosphere (and there are just as many or more studies out there proving the efficacy of essential oils).

- **The group chattering is a very small, very loud group.** They remind me of that 5% of guys that come through our program that cause all the tension there. The difference is that I'm sure the chatter on the Internet is less than 5% of the sum total of the total information about YL that's out there. Yes, it often comes up first when you do a Google search, but I could get *any* of my stuff to come up first, too, for a low fee paid to Google and other search engines for every click-through.

- **The "everybody is jumping on the bandwagon" argument they use is foolish**. A few Internet haters have actually used the "bandwagon" argument as a reason *not* to use the oils. It's their version of *"If everybody jumped off a cliff, would you?"* I just might jump if the cliff was 4-5 feet high. Or if my kid was sick and his remedy was at the bottom. Or if there was a pile of money at the bottom. Face it: we bandwagon *good* things all the time. If something is really good, we *hope* that people will bandwagon the thing. Every time a preacher declares truth, he's *praying* for a bandwagon.

- **I don't know those Internet haters**, so I don't have any reason to trust them, anyway. Nor do you.

And think about this: **didn't Jesus say you would know them by their fruit?**[12] Not by their excessive words or self-proclaimed greatest hits version of themselves? Not by their lack of naysayers.

In a world that blogs about *any* action the Pope takes (good or bad) *while* simultaneously nit-picking what celebrities wore to the Oscars, would it surprise you that there is some chatter out there about Young Living?

The Apostle Paul himself had a thorn in the flesh.[13] That doesn't make me want to "give up" on or abandon The Gospel, though, in the same way that some people read a little negativity and want to abandon the hope and healing offered through essential oils!

I've concluded that Gary probably doesn't respond to any of the chatter for a few reasons. First, the chatter would never stop. He would spend all of his time arguing about this and that or the other. Second, that's not his mission- to try to appease people who will never like him. **His focus is to learn about the plants God has given us stewardship over- and to use them in the best possible way to bring health and healing and wholeness**. So, my guess is that he just quietly lets it go and does his thing.

Is it hurtful to know others are stabbing you in the back? *Yes.*

Can you do anything about it? *No.*

---

[12] Matthew 7:15-20

[13] 2 Corinthians 12:7

Conclusion: Simply rise above it and move on. Besides, Proverbs says, "Argue with a fool and you'll never win."[14] So why waste the time?

Here's the truth, too: even if Gary was the chump they portray him to be (which he's clearly not), the oils still work. I'd take the health benefits from them anyway. And the reality is that Gary is a wonderful man.

> Gary didn't start distilling oils in order to create a business, he started distilling oils in order to heal himself.

Bottom line: I'm not going to be distracted by a hater. Especially if the hater has no vested interest in me or the person he's hating on. You shouldn't either.

Like a legend

I've personally met Gary. And I've watched him interact with other people. He's everything his staff says- and *more*- and nothing the Internet haters say.

I've shaken his hand a few times (calloused, from years of working as a logger and repeated trips into the field *even now* as the CEO of a major corporation). I've hugged him. He's embraced me. I decided the first time I saw him that **he is larger than life in a humble way. That, and his love is loud and colossally big.**

He hugged just about everyone at that event in Hawaii, in fact. He and Mary both did. They genuinely love people and *adore* hearing their stories of overcoming disease and debt alike.

I've watched him stand in place while time stood still as a line of dozens and dozens of people get their picture taken with him. I've seen him listen as intently and sincerely- and be emotionally moved by the first person's story of gratitude all the way through to the last person speaking.

"How old are you?" I asked him, about the second time I met him. We were on the balcony at his suite in Hawaii. He had invited the "Top 10" winners in the *Drive to Win* promotion to his place for dinner.

---

[14] My paraphrase. Proverbs 26:4 reads: "When arguing with fools, don't answer their foolish arguments, or you will become as foolish as they are" (New Living Translation).

Until that trip, I was probably a pseudo-skeptic about Young Living. Not a skeptic about the oils, but just a *"Is this too good to be true?"* type of questioner about the hype and hoopla that seemed to surround everything. That changed on the trip.

Last August, right after Cristy enrolled as a distributor for Young Living, the corporate office announced the *Drive to Win* contest. Distributors received points for things like enrolling new members, setting people up on Essential Rewards, and helping the members under her also enroll other members.

Cristy heard about the contest after someone in her upline messaged her: "Look at the leaderboard- you're on it!" We were like 37th or so. That meant *she* would win an all expense paid trip, but I would have to pay to go.

She had some alone time in the shower one day (that's the only alone time you get with nine kids) and prayed, "Lord, I would love to go… and I would love to be in the Top 10!" A top ten win would secure a place for her and a guest- *all expenses paid*. That would mean we could both go free of charge!

She says that He assured her it was done. She would be going. I heard stories about people stressing and "working it" hard to get atop the leader board. Cristy never did that. She was chill the entire time. She heard from the Lord and resolved He would get her a ticket for two.

Turns out, He did.

I watched her name bump up the list for the next months until, alas, there we were in Hawaii- standing on Gary's balcony. That's when I had asked Gary how old he was…

"Sixty-five," he offered with a slight smile.

"You look great for sixty-five," I replied.

He grinned. Then- "I don't feel it. My back and my arms and my body got whacked from years of logging and other little adventures," he laughed.

When I heard about his 1973 paralyzing logging accident (a tree fell and struck him violently on the head, rendering him unable to walk- and likely unable to ever do so), I decided he might be a living legend. Apparently, he was wheelchair bound with no hope for walking again. Ever. It was his search for alternative paths of healing, after modern medicine had done all it could do, that led him to the oils.[15]

Gary writes, "Within two years, I went from a wheelchair to a walker, to crutches, and then to walking, but not without considerable pain."[16] He could only walk short distances after that, but found himself walking without pain after using higher grade essential oils. It was at this point that the "quality issue" became a factor. This continues to be a driving force in the Young Living culture. Quite simply: *better quality is better.*

A week after using the oils, he began jogging. In 1986, he entered a marathon and placed 60th out of 970 runners. His health was back.

> His focus is to learn about the plants God has given us stewardship over- and to use them in the best possible way to bring health and healing and wholeness.

Notice, though, **Gary didn't start distilling oils in order to create a business, he started distilling oils in order to heal himself.**

It's the same story I heard over and over that week in Hawaii from distributors themselves- I don't know of *a single one* that got into Young Living in order to make money. Every person I heard from testified that they began using the oils… and the business opportunity grew from there.[17]

Oddly enough, it was while I was doing some research about Quack Watch for this book that I uncovered a few other obscure facts about Gary.[18] Facts like he has a weightlifting and backpacking regimen. He lifted enough weights to place first in the 2002 Western States Fitness Contest. He was in his mid-50s then- and came back to take second place the following year.[19]

Apparently, Gary jousts competitively, also. While searching background info for this book, I learned somewhere that Gary took second in the 2003 World Championship Jousting Association's International Dragon's Lair Jousting

---

[15] Gary recounts this in his book *Aromatherapy: The Essential Beginning,* an excellent intro to essential oils.

[16] Page 2 of *An Introduction to Young Living Essential Oils,* by D. Gary Young.

[17] Side note: this is one of the factors that distinguishes Young Living from a pyramid scheme. In a pyramid scheme, people push profits- not *products.* And people sign up for profits- not *products.*

[18] As mentioned before, this info didn't make the final cut of the book. It's irrelevant.

[19] This contest was hosted by the National Physique Committee.

Tournament… and fifth place in the light armor division. I didn't even know such things existed. Apparently YL does, because there's a full fledged jousting arena at the corporate headquarters!

And, of course, like all legends, Gary is *silent* about the exploits. He tells me his back is out of whack from logging. I sense there's more to it. But Paul Bunyan never bragged about his blue ox and Johnny Appleseed never talked about anything more than just planting those fruit trees.

The people in the room

We moved the furniture and the food into Gary's dining room from the spacious balcony that night, shortly after I asked him about his age. It had begun to rain just as we were going around the circle of twenty or so people, at Gary's request, sharing our version of how we got involved in Young Living. So in went the massive trays of pineapples and other fruits, along with too-many-to-count bottles of Ningxia Red. One thing I remember about that week was that Ningxia Red was served with every meal- all you can drink. Even for breakfast.

"Tell us about yourself," Gary instructed the crowd. It was the Top 10, the group who won the all expenses paid trip for two. "Tell us all how you ended up becoming involved with Young Living." He's quiet and unhurried when he speaks, whether he's addressing a large crowd or a single person.

We heard from the Canadian couple- the husband's back had given out after a botched back surgery a few years ago.

"Six months ago it was impossible for me to walk like I did today," he told us, referring to the hiking around the hills of the Sandalwood farms we had visited earlier in the day. "I could barely stand to wash the dishes for thirty minutes or so after dinner and would be exhausted…overcome with pain." He took the oils his wife suggested and started getting better, almost instantly. The healing process began instantly. "I feel like I have my life back," he said.

The following day he was with us on a zip line trip. I asked him afterwards how he felt, knowing that the jarring from jumping full weight into line would certainly rattle your spine if you had *any* tenderness there at all.

"I felt awesome," he said. It was the same thing he told that group that night. "Our involvement in Young Living has changed our outlook financially and physically…"

By the way, I watched Gary talk to this guy, also named Gary, and his wife when no one was watching. On the balcony. Just the three of them. They were discussing protocol for one of their kids that faces a major medical situation. I watched Gary stand with them patiently... unmoved by the time it took to delicately talk through scenario after scenario... as a father would talk to his own grown children about their young son- one he would love as his own grandson. He was like that with everyone there.

As we went around the circle, we heard from the couple with the "failed" business. Heidi explained that a payroll company had collected tax money from them then pocketed the money instead of paying those taxes. When the government came collecting, they figured out a way to pay.

> Like every other person it the room, *we never signed up with Young Living for the business opportunity...*

Five years later, the economy tanked and caught them off-guard. There wasn't another nest egg, like they had when the tax issue came up. They sold everything they had- down to the bare walls. They cashed-out their retirement plans and even had to live off their young kids' savings accounts.

"We sold it all and moved 3,000 miles away from South Carolina to Canada," she explained.

Her husband, tall, handsome, and slender... a builder... grinned with the kind of pleasant delight you use to communicate when you've overcome a massive hurdle that you knew was an oncoming freight train.

Heidi looked at him and told us, "He moved his business all the way to another country. We re-started. A do over."

Just 18 months into her work as a Distributor, his business is booming- and so is hers. "We've never been so excited about the future," they said. For the first time in a long time, they had a new lease on life. And that lease was very good.

We heard from the couple who both found themselves without employment just before getting married. The man, tall and sharp, wisecracked as to how he might approach his then fiancé's father, explaining how he might provide for his daughter one day. That day was *now*.

His wife told us how she, a news anchor, had ulcers in her mouth. Fifteen or twenty of them. It affected how she could talk, which affected her paycheck.

When work wasn't coming, success in Young Living did. Now the couple, expecting their first child any day now, is financially free.

We heard from the chiropractor. The oils had changed his business practices. As many people were coming to him and his wife for the oils as were coming for adjustments and alignments. He was thrilled.

From the acupuncturist. He was quite skilled, but had started seeing profound improvements in his patients, since incorporating Young Living into his practice. He proudly brought his dad on the trip, also a beautiful man.

From the minister who had been sick for years. She was now walking in healing and proclaiming a message to others that she would tell us several times over the weekend: "I really believe God wants people well... He has an amazing destiny for everyone, but they can't walk in that destiny if they're sick in bed."

Oh, her first words to the group were, "*I can't believe this is my life*... that this is actually my life..."

Joseph, Gary's 10 year-old son, regularly kept the conversation moving from one person to the next. He's full of life- in a boyish sort of way. He's a kid that takes everything in, absorbs it all, and then let's it out. I imagine that he and his older brother will one day be trekking with Gary in remote places of the earth, digging roots, examining leaves, and studying the science behind it all. For now, he's 110% boy.

"What place were you in the contest?" Joseph asked each person as they concluded their story for the circle of new friends.

Eventually, we started introducing ourselves by number and name. Joseph seemed pleased.

Then it was our turn to talk. We were number *eight*.

I just wanted to get out of the house

"I just wanted to get out of the house, one night," Cristy confessed. She explained that we had been using essential oils for years- of other brands. Then- "We have nine kids, and it had *already* been one of those weeks!"

The women in the room laughed. Somehow, the husbands... well, we all knew that somehow we contribute to those weeks.

"A friend invited me to a restaurant on the other side of town," she continued. "I went there and I had already eaten at home, so I ordered water. I sat in that back conference room of the restaurant and there wasn't even a live teacher. Crystal Burchfield was teaching through a speakerphone that was sitting in the middle of the table."

Crystal is Verick's wife. You'll meet him later in the book. They were in Hawaii, too, just not in the room. They weren't in the Top 10, but a lot of us standing in the Young's suite that night made it there *because of Crystal*- her business had taken off and she had introduced others who introduced others who introduced us. And they had resourced their team incredibly well.

"I had been using essential oils for years," my wife relayed. "I had even heard of Young Living before- quite a few years ago." She outlined a few ways in which the oils had blessed us…

- Our kids don't get the flu when it runs through the city, because they gargle or drink Thieves.

- Judah sleeps extremely well because he puts Peace & Calming on his feet every evening before bed.

- We healed sunburns with Lavender at the beach this past summer.

- Cristy swears that I don't snore when she rubs Valor on my spine. I've not known myself to snore- though *she has assured me* that I sleep right through it every time, even though it sounds like an indoor hurricane.

Like every other person it the room, *we never signed up with Young Living for the business opportunity*. Cristy explained that amid more sympathetic chuckles and grins that all acknowledged, "We thought that, too…"

The eccentric Frenchman

The circle concluded with Travis, who is one of the top execs, and then Gary. Travis said a few words about how our grateful attitudes were so encouraging- and how that grace was contagious.

Then it was Gary's turn. We had been standing in that circle for about half an hour, but time stood still and no one seemed to care.

"I remember looking for a man for five years," Gary told us. That's how he launched into the story about the eccentric Frenchman. "His name was Mr. Vue."

He travelled to France to look for him and was unsuccessful. Then he asked around and travelled again. No luck. And again and again. And again.

"Finally," Gary told us, "I found a friend who knew him and agreed to invite him over to dinner. He would invite me, too, and then we would be able to talk."

Gary wanted to learn and soak up all you could about distilling from this mysterious Mr. Vue. Apparently, Vue was *the* expert in the field. If you were going to learn about distilling, *he* was the best place to go.

Gary explained that in France dinner goes differently than in America. "You have an appetizer and talk for 20 or 30 minutes," he said. "Then they take those plates and bring out salads. You talk for 30 more minutes or so…"

...this was a pivotal moment. *It was more than just a question…*

It dawned on me that in the time we usually pound down a meal and sit back in front of the television or our computers, they hadn't *really* even started the meal.

"Someone brings out breads and cheeses… and then a main course. There's 30 more minutes of talking and then more wine and more food… Then they clear all of those plates and bring you a desert. Maybe more wine, maybe more coffee, definitely lots of conversation…"

He estimated that if you were making fast time, you would wrap it in 2.5 or 3 hours.

"I was sitting across the table from my friend," Gary said, diagramming the table in mid-air with his hands, there for all of us in the circle to see. "Mr. Vue was sitting immediately to my left and to my friend's right- at the end of the table."

Then he hit us with the oddity of the night- "The two of them spoke in French the entire evening. Mr. Vue never even made eye contact with me. I just talked to my friend's wife. She was sitting on the other side of him, caddy-cornered to me."

Gary continued, "As things were wrapping up, and I sensed my opportunity to learn from this man had slipped away, he fervently grabbed me on the forearm, clenching it firmly. He looked me square in the eyes, his eyes staring through me, deep into my soul. Then he asked me in a deep European accent, 'Mistah Gary, *what are essential oils to you…?'*"

"I had no idea that he understand *any* English at all," Gary told us. "He hadn't used any the whole time we were eating. And there he was, putting the question of the night on the table. This man had been listening to me talk to my friend's wife the entire meal. Somehow, I knew, too… in the way he said that question… and in the way he was holding my arm… that this was a pivotal moment. *It was more than just a question…*"

Gary told us that he quickly gathered his thoughts and then relayed the first thing that came to mind, hoping that he came out the right way and was heard in the right way: "Essentials oils, Sir, are the closet thing to God we have on this planet."

He sunk back in his chair. Time stopped. It was like those times in the movies when something's about to happen and the silence gets loud and you only hear the clocks tick.

Then, immediately, Mr. Vue pointed towards the ceiling and exclaimed, "You are exactly right!"

> Essentials oils… are the closet thing to God we have on this planet.

With that, Vue excused himself, stood up, gave a courtesy, "I have to go, it's getting late," and pushed his chair back beneath the table.

Gary and the host went to walk him out, Gary somewhat certain his opportunity was walking out the door. As he waited in the living room, leaning his head over the mantle of the fireplace, the host walked Vue to the car.

"Tough night," he told Gary, pulling the door behind him.

Gary nodded in agreement and stood there, collecting his thoughts. Retracing steps. Replaying how he'd tried to track Vue down for five years. It had all come to this. One question. One answer. He was *right*. But the man still walked out the door.

The host returned a moment later. "You should go to bed, Gary… it's getting late."

Gary agreed, thinking maybe sleep was the best way to bury that lengthy chapter of his life.

Then the host tapped him on the arm, locked eyes with him, and told him, "You have a long day ahead of you. Mr. Vue wants you on the mountain with him bright and early in the morning!"

Gary says he floated up the landing to his room. He slept and yet didn't sleep all in one that night. The dream was going to come true.

Turns out, he worked with Mr. Vue and began learning the distillation process. The first week or so, Gary was told to sleep outside in a small shed near the distiller. It was his job to keep the fire burning and the distiller hot.

Bit by bit, **he learned more and more, literally starting from the bottom.** Vue eventually offered him use of the house, forging a relationship that still exists with Vue's wife and family today- several years after the eccentric Frenchman has died. When in France, they still visit and often stay with that family, back where it all began.

Gary told them his dreams of having lavender fields in America, of growing his own crops and distilling them one day with his own machines. When he first opened the fields, he invited Vue to the Grand Opening.

Vue offered him what he still believes to be one of the highest compliments he's received. "Ah… Gary… yes… beautiful. Now the student has become the teacher, and the teacher is the student."

Gary teared-up as he communicated the story, showing not only how important the entire thing was to his life path, but how relationally invested his life was with the eccentric Frenchman.

People before products and profits

Mary arrived in Hawaii later that evening, so we didn't meet her until the following day. I'll tell you more about that conversation later, because she said a few things that helped the idea of multilevel marketing "click" for me. Anyway, she asked how we were enjoying ourselves and what we thought about the company, since Cristy and I were relatively new…

"Your husband is fabulous," I told her. "He shared his story about Mr. Vue and I could sense his love for him… It dawned on me after he told us the story that he's probably communicated it *thousands* of times by now. It's been over twenty years. And yet he is *still* moved by it. He really loves people…"

She confirmed my first impressions- that Gary genuinely loves prop le and that he loves them deeply.

I told her something else I learned, "You all tell us that the products are more important than the profits- and that if you take care of the products that the profits will come and you'll be able to stay in business…"

"Yes," she told me, with a smile that permanently fills her youthful face. "We really believe that."

And they do. Young Living manages their own farms and contracts with others when necessary. Yet they still maintain rigorous standards and quality controls. They'll throw millions of dollars of products in the trash before taking something that would simply "pass the muster" to market. The bottom line could be higher, but Gary constantly invests in the fields and in researching better ways to do things.[20]

I continued, "Mary, I don't know that the products are the most important thing to you all… I was there last night in that room. I saw the affection your husband had for the people he had just met this week. I saw him unhurried with each of them. He recorded multiple videos for us to send to our friends, congratulating them on their progress in their businesses. He didn't rush any of it. I've seen him interact with his staff here and how he loves them…He was constantly in the moment…"

> The most important thing… did not seem to be the products. The most important thing is the people… I bet that if Gary had to choose between the products and the people, he would quit tomorrow and keep the people.

Then I gave her my assessment. "The most important thing to your husband did not seem to be the products. The most important thing is the people." As she nodded in agreement, I added, "I bet that if Gary had to choose between the products and the people, he would quit tomorrow and keep the people…"

---

[20] Read more about the Seed to Seal process later in the book.

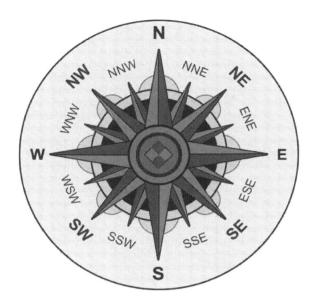

01: Direction: get started

Action steps

☐ Here's my suggestion: *Go on a media fast for about two weeks.*

> **Main idea:** Some things that seem too good to be true are actually good and true.

Don't read the newspaper (someone at the office will tell you if anything important happens, trust me). Limit your time on FaceBook (gasp!).[21] Chunk the reality shows and the other stuff on TV and Netflix. *Just for a few days.* Nothing in any of those places in going to change your life. None of it. **Instead of spending the time there, spend the time doing a bit of reconnaissance about Young Living and your wife's business.** Read some of the articles and book chapters I'll reference in this book, listen to a few

---

[21] One of the ironies of this is that I'm going to send you right back to FaceBook in a few chapters to connect with some guys. It will be way better than mindlessly scrolling through the timeline, though.

of the podcasts, and let her tell you something about a few of the oils. Just for 2-3 weeks, alright?

☐ By the way, in the "Want to know more?" section in each of these chapters throughout the book, I'll provide you with that info. If you find something on your own that I haven't included that you think may be helpful, send it to me and I'll post it for other guys to pick up on the next edit.

☐ Also, I've placed links to all of this info on my blog: www.TheHusbandsFieldGuide.com will take you to the page dedicated to this info.

Want to know more?

☐ Read:

   ☐ "What is Aromatherapy?" Chapter 1 in *An Introduction to Young Living Essential Oils*, by D. Gary Young

   ☐ "Young Living Farms," Chapter 4 in *An Introduction to Young Living Essential Oils*, by D. Gary Young

☐ Listen:

   ☐ To the relevant chapter of the audiobook

☐ Search:

   ☐ Go to Young Living's website and look around (www.YoungLiving.com). You may want to start on the "About" page, then follow a few links about the founder: https://www.youngliving.com/en_US/company/about .

   ☐ Gary Young has a blog where he posts about once a week. You can find it here: www.DGaryYoung.com .

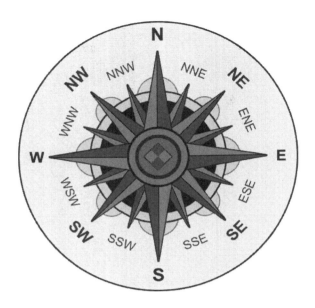

01: Take these meds forever, or... / Marty's story

I am an active happily married 40-year old who has a young family who always keep me on the run. I love playing golf but have a demanding job so I work about 50 hours a week. I sneak a round of golf or the range in every chance I get. That is my out, my way to relieve stress.

Marty Harbert has been married to Tiffany over 15 years. They have two children, a boy and a girl. Tiffany has been a distributor with Young Living since October 2013.

I always heard that your body falls apart when you turn 40. Around July of 2013 right after my birthday, I began to think that might be true. I started noticing my ankles were sore. I had played golf recently and had been working in the yard, so I assumed I was feeling pain due to the activity.

I popped some Ibuprofen and brushed it off.

My ankles continued to hurt, though- some days worse than others. Ibuprofen kept my pain at bay and I was able to get through the day without thinking much about it. It was happening. I was falling apart at 40.

Days passed and my wife asked how my ankles were doing. I replied they felt somewhat better but my elbows were now hurting. Again, I disregarded the pain, assuming it was somehow golf related- or that I had pulled something doing who knows what.

It did get a little better when I took Ibuprofen to ease the pain.

But just when I thought it was resolving itself and I was on the mend, my knees began hurting. Then the elbow pain came back. A few weeks later my ankles started to swell. The bottoms of my feet hurt so bad I just knew I had planters fasciitis. All was helped with Ibuprofen, but I found I needed to take several a day to get through the pain.

I started researching and found out I might be overdosing on Vitamin C. I lowered my daily intake to see if that would help with my pain. I was hoping that was my answer since it was a simple fix.

See, I don't like Doctors and I don't like going to them to be put on medication. Ironic, I know, with my daily regimen of Ibuprofen. I never have and I really don't like taking OTC meds but I hurt so bad I had to — a couple times a day— to work through the pain.

The pain grew into stiffness and different joints seem to be affected at different times. Each morning I would wake up and the pain and stiffness would worsen.

By early fall, I could barely get out of bed in the morning. I felt 90 years old. It took about 15 minutes for me to be able to walk well at all.

I remember thinking 40 was "old" until I approached that gleaming age and found out it wasn't old at all. Some of you know the drill- when you're a kid, you feel like you're 40-year old Mom is ancient. Then you get there yourself and you think, "I've still got it. I'm good..."

I was like that, until my body started falling apart. Then my mind changed quickly. My wife and I, of course, thought the worst, so I broke down and made an appointment with a Doctor of Internal Medicine.

He ran every test he could on me, but nothing really stood out. I felt lucky that nothing pointed to cancer or anything incurable.

Since the doctor didn't find anything wrong with me, he sent me to a rheumatologist as my next step. We were at the point where we had to start ruling out other ailments.

The rheumatologist did some tests, asked a series of questions, and basically said my symptoms were arthritic-type symptoms but that my condition pointed to spinal neuropathy. The rheumatologist also said my pain stemmed from the spine- odd because my spine didn't necessarily hurt, but all my pain was allegedly caused from the spinal neuropathy.

I had a back surgery in 2003 and had a metal plate inserted. Wondering if this had anything to do with my now problems I listened to the new doctor and answered all his questions. He pretty much said that there was a prescription he could write me to aid with the pain and should knock it down enough to be comfortable. That was what the doctor was going for- tolerating and managing the pain, not necessarily eliminating the cause.

I asked him, "Is something I will have to take the rest of my life?"

He replied, "Do you want to hurt the rest of your life?"

I didn't, I told him. That's why I was there- to not hurt anymore.

"If not then I suggest you take the prescription," the doctor said.

Not happy with this answer I still had to know that his diagnosis was correct, so I took the medication for the 2 weeks he prescribed. Now, it did help with the pain after a day or two of it getting into my system. I continued through to the entire 2 weeks and was satisfied that he was correct.

However, I was not satisfied with the "take this for the rest of your life if you don't want to live in pain" attitude. Not to mention my kidneys were starting to manifest a bit of pain of their own.

My wife and I started researching all the side effects and learned that liver and kidney damage were possibilities with long term use. Since my kidneys had already started hurting with use, my attention was arrested.

This lit a fire under my wife. She went on a hunt and found Young Living through Cristy, a high school friend. She trusted Cristy, did a little research and, then decided this was worth a try.

After hours of research, she placed an order for the kit and a few other oils. We knew this was going to be "trial and error" thing, but Tiffany she was determined. She tried several oils topically with some results, but I had not found the oil- or oils- to knock back my pain and discomfort.

In November, I started Lemongrass and Clove, 3 drops of each in a capsule, twice a day. This seemed to help me tremendously. After 2 weeks I felt like this was my combo.

We learned the essential oils target the receptor cells for repair, so we began using Copaiba down my spine twice a day. For as long as I can remember I have had a spot on the bottom of my feet that felt like a bruise. My wife showed me the Vita Flex chart and I discovered the place on the bottom of my foot was exactly where the spine was located. So she added the Copaiba to my feet at night on the Vita Flex point for the spine. Within a day, that place no longer hurt and I was completely amazed.

We do this regimen daily- have been doing it since the middle of November. I stopped using the prescription and have now been prescription free since the end of November, just two weeks after the oil regimen began. I have no pain, no discomfort, no swelling.

I have started playing golf again, and I am actively working out. It is as if nothing was ever wrong with me. The oils are truly amazing, and I am very thankful for my wife taking on the initiative to find a natural remedy.

- Marty Harbert, Tiffany's husband

Marty's story

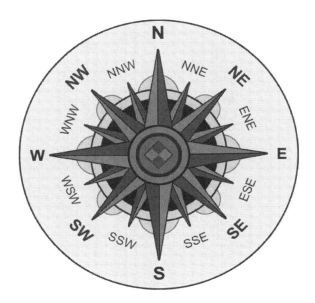

02: The trees are for the healing of the nations

I was running the last morning we were in Hawaii. Remember, I decided to start losing the extra thirty pounds? That was the day I started. The following verse perked in my mind:

Then he showed me a river of the water of life, clear as crystal, coming from the throne of God and of the Lamb, in the middle of its street. On either side of the river was the tree of life, bearing twelve kinds of fruit, yielding its fruit every month; and **the leaves of the tree were for the healing of the nations.**[22]

> **The main idea:** Let's embrace new technologies and not overlook anything that might be helpful for us. At the same time, let's not forget the oldest and purest solutions of all.

---

[22] Revelation 22:1-2 (NIV, emphasis mine).

The prophet Ezekiel foresaw this thousands of years before John, who wrote that verse during a vision of his own:

> *Fruit trees of all kinds will grow on both banks of the river. Their leaves will not wither, nor will their fruit fail. Every month they will bear fruit, because the water from the sanctuary flows to them. Their fruit will serve for food and **their leaves for healing.**[23]*

Here's my view: things are getting *better*- not worse. A lot of people are certain that the world is falling apart, that everyone is evil, and that literally any moment we're all doomed. If you watch the evening news, they'll skip telling you about all of the incredible things people are doing and confirm these worst suspicions.

Yes, sin happened and The Fall came. And bad things still occur. Every day. I understand first hand. I see it at my "real job" every day. Yet, Jesus restored all things by shedding His blood on the Cross. *All things*. Peter preached about the restoration of *everything*.[24] Moses did, too- long before Peter.[25] I don't have time to get into it over a few short pages, but the word for salvation that is used in the Bible, *sozo*, means far more than just the forgiveness of sins. It means forgiveness, healing, provision, freedom…[26] Jesus came to hit a reset button on everything that sin caused.

Remember, in the Garden of Eden, God gave Adam and Eve stewardship over *everything*. In a real sense, when we get back to the basics of stewarding the plants that He created- all of which were created good- we are getting back to one of the core purposes we had in the very beginning.

I didn't learn this in seminary

Gary tells a story about the real Indiana Jones. Yes, turns out George Lucas based this character on several real life characters who were as smart and

---

[23] Ezekiel 47:12 (NIV, emphasis added).

[24] Acts 3:21.

[25] See Deuteronomy 30:3-13.

[26] See "Salvation is everything Jesus came to do," taught 7/14/13 at The Grace Church, http://thegracechurchmedia.wordpress.com/2013/07/14/supernatural-1-salvation-is-everything-jesus-came-to-do/, accessed 3/4/2014.

physically adventurous as the Harrison Ford version you saw on the big screen.[27]

"I think Jesus made multiple trips to Egypt throughout His life," Gary's story goes. "Even the Bible tells us that there is a lot He did that wouldn't fit in the Bible. In just the 40 or 50 pages of the Gospels you don't have His entire life."

Indeed, John tells us that if everything Jesus did was written down, that "the world could not contain all of the books."[28] Perhaps the disciple is exaggerating a bit, but he gives you a pretty good idea that Jesus did *a whole lot more* than just what's in the Bible.

"Some historians believe Jesus made *five* trips to Egypt," Gary explains. "You read about the one when Joseph and Mary fled from Herod when Jesus was young, shortly after the wise men came to see them..."[29]

> "The fact that gold reserves were left behind attests to the value of the the precious oils that were once inside..."

Gary believes that Jesus learned about essential oils during those subsequent trips. In fact, in his introductory book to essential oils he writes that "Some say essential oils were first used in China or India. But my research indicates that the Egyptians were first to discover the therapeutic potential of essential oils. The Egyptians created fragrances for personal use as well as for ritualistic and ceremonial use in temples and pyramids."[30]

He explains that an almost 900-foot long papyrus was discovered in 1817. That's a scroll that unrolls the length of three football fields. I'm not an Auburn fan (I pull for the Tide, actually), but that's 9 of the "Kick 6" returned failed field goal attempts that dashed Alabama's hopes for a three-peat.[31] In other words, that's a lot of information.

---

[27] http://en.wikipedia.org/wiki/Indiana_Jones , read the sections on "Character description and formation" and "Origins and inspirations."

[28] John 21:25

[29] Matthew 2:13f.

[30] Gary Young, *An Introduction to Young Living Essential Oils*, p3.

[31] http://en.wikipedia.org/wiki/Kick_Bama_Kick, accessed 03-20-2014.

The info on the scroll dates back to 1500 years before the time of Christ. "It was called a medicinal scroll."[32] Noting the medicines on that scroll: "It mentioned over 800 herbal prescriptions and remedies."[33] All *natural*. Organic. Like the Garden of Eden.

Here's where the Indiana Jones part comes in: King Tut's tomb was opened and explored in 1922. The crew that mined the tombs discovered 50 alabaster jars, each designed to hold approximately 7 liters of oil. Indeed, "well before the time of Christ, the ancient Egyptians collected essential oils and placed them in alabaster vessels... In 1922, when King Tutankhamen's tomb was opened, some 50 alabaster jars designed to hold 350 liters of oil were discovered."[34] Some contained residue that revealed the original contents; others were completely plundered. **The fact that gold reserves were left behind attests to the value of the the precious oils that were once inside.**[35]

Though you may initially react at the thought that Jesus "learned" more information than what you might have thought He already knew, remember that the Bible tells us that He "grew in wisdom and in stature

> What does it mean that He grew in wisdom, though? ... *Did this include the use of essential oils?*

and in favor with God and man."[36] In other words, Jesus *changed* as He aged.

Jesus grew in stature- He developed physically in the same manner every other baby boy has grown through adolescence into adulthood.

He also grew relationally- the first one mentioned ("favor with God") is confusing, because we read in the Bible that He and the Father are one.[37] Perhaps He learned to walk with a more thorough awareness of that relationship. Jesus also learned to relate well with those around Him. He learned the dynamics of relationships and human interaction firsthand.

---

[32] Gary Young, *An Introduction to Young Living Essential Oils*, p3.

[33] Gary Young, *An Introduction to Young Living Essential Oils*, p3.

[34] *Essential Oils Pocket Reference*, p4.

[35] Gary Young, *An Introduction to Young Living Essential Oils*, p3, emphasis mine. Gary writes that "Kings would barter and buy land, gold, and slaves with their crudely extracted oils because they were more valuable than gold" (p3).

[36] Luke 2:52

[37] John 10:30

What does it mean that He grew in wisdom, though? Perhaps, Jesus grew in the practical application of everyday things. Did this include everyday skills like carpentry, that He would learn from His father, Joseph? And wouldn't it include learning to buy, trade, or sell His skill set and wares? Did He learn how to cleanse a wound during his long, hard days or how to bandage/set a broken bone? *Did this include the use of essential oils?*

I earned my Master's of Divinity (M.Div.) from Baylor University in 1999.[38] During my seminary days, I never read or heard anything about any of what I've just written. Of course, Baylor is a Baptist school- a more liberal one than some of the fundamentalist versions that smatter the South, but still very Biblically conservative. We never even discussed anointing oil, even though that concept appears throughout the Bible. We left oils, waving banners, and extended altar calls in which people "fall out" to the Charismatics and Pentecostals.

Jesus changed / Luke 2:52

Wisdom	Jesus grew in the practical application of everyday things. *Did this include the use of essential oils?*
Stature	Jesus developed physically in the same manner every other baby boy has grown through adolescence into adulthood.
Favor with God	Jesus grew relationally. This first one is confusing, because we read in the Bible that He and the Father are one. Perhaps He learned to walk with a more thorough awareness of that relationship.
Favor with man	Jesus learned to relate well with those around Him. He learned the dynamics of relationships and human interaction firsthand.

From Egypt to The Tabernacle?

All throughout the Old Testament, particularly in the time of Moses, we see the prominence of essential oils. There are well over 200 references.[39] The Egyptian

---

[38] George W. Truett Theological Seminary is the name of the seminary at Baylor in Waco, Texas.

[39] *Essential Oils Pocket Reference*, p6, 10-14.

connection makes sense when you remember that Moses was steeped in Egyptian tradition. He was a true "prince of Egypt" and raised as such, until he fled for his life after killing a fellow Egyptian in the fields.[40]

The Lord gave very specific instructions, for instance, about the building of the Tabernacle, the furniture and relics that were to be placed inside, and the adornment of the priests who would administer specific sacrifices. He was clear, too, that those priests were to be anointed with a *specific* blend of essential oils which He relayed to Moses:

> He was clear, too, that those priests were to be anointed with a *specific* blend of essential oils which He relayed to Moses.

Take the finest spices: of liquid myrrh 500 shekels, and of sweet-smelling cinnamon half as much, that is, 250, and 250 of aromatic cane, and 500 of cassia, according to the shekel of the sanctuary, and a hin of olive oil. And you shall make of these a sacred anointing oil blended as by the perfumer; it shall be a holy anointing oil.[41]

For mathematic purposes, 500 shekels is about one gallon.[42] In effect, Moses was blending the following:

- Myrrh- 1 gallon (500 shekels)

- Cinnamon- 1/2 gallon (250 shekels)

- Calamus- 1/2 gallon (250 shekels)

- Cassia- 1 gallon (500 shekels)

- Olive oil- about 1 & 1/3 gallons ("a hin" is slightly larger)

When complete, he had almost a five gallon bucket of anointing oil. If they didn't ration it when applying the anointing oil, it would *drench* the man being anointed.

Consider this passage from Psalm 133:1-3[43]:

---

[40] Exodus 2:12f.

[41] Exodus 30:23-25, English Standard Version.

[42] See *Essential Oils Pocket Reference*, pp6-7.

[43] Psalm 133:1-3, English Standard Version, emphasis added.

> *Behold, how good and pleasant it is*
> *when brothers dwell in unity!*
>
> *It is like the precious oil* **on the head,**
> **running down on the beard,**
> *on the beard of Aaron,*
> **running down on the collar of his robes***!*
>
> *It is like the dew of Hermon,*
> *which falls on the mountains of Zion!*
> *For there the Lord has commanded the blessing,*
> *life forevermore.*

Notice that the oil flows down the robes as it falls off the priest's head, fills his beard, and hits the collar. That's *a lot* of oil!

There were actually people in ancient Israel whose job it was to maintain the stock of anointing- and other- oils. They were known as "apothecaries" or "perfumers."[44] My guess is that most of them were of the priestly class.

Keep in mind that priests in that culture were likely stout and strong-like cowboys. They had to maneuver live animals onto the altar to be sacrificed. In other words, these perfumers weren't like the guy

> Does this make the Bible stories less dramatic, less supernatural? *Not at all.*

that walks around spritzing you with cologne or giving you sample perfume cards in the mall. They were tough.

You see them building the stone wall around the city with Nehemiah after the exile, even. He writes, "Hannaniah, one of the *perfumers*, made repairs."[45] Building the wall was intense physically not only because of the labor, but also because the men had to defend themselves from invaders while they built. The oil guys, AKA perfumers, were there.

Still not convinced that essential oils are in the Bible? Let me introduce you to Korah. He's is one of the guys who led a rebellion against Moses in the

---

[44] See 1 Chronicles 9:30, as well as page 65 of *Healing Oils of the Bible.*

[45] See Nehemiah 3:8, New King James Version, emphasis mine.

wilderness. Moses told everyone to step away from him, then the earth opened up and swallowed him whole- a massive sink hole appeared out of nowhere.[46]

You would *think* that everyone would get the message- don't argue against the Lord's anointed. But, alas, they were prideful. Korah's rebellion in large part had been based around the notion of "What makes Moses so special?" I suppose others still wanted to know.

Immediately after Korah was swallowed by the earth, people started complaining to Moses about Moses' own leadership. Again.

So a plague broke out and Aaron, instructed by God, came to the rescue.[47] If you read the story you'll notice he did something that seemed strange: he fumigated the area with an aromatic smoke, using a blend of frankincense, galbanum, onycha, and myrrh.

Sure, the Lord was honored by their obedience, but did you know that galbanum's (the second oil) frequency is increased (it's therapeutic affects are made stronger) when added to frankincense? And, it is known to elevate the mind, "helping to overcome stress and despair."[48]

Here's a bit of Old Testament irony: Joseph (the boy with the coat of many colors who was detested by his brothers) was sold to a group of essential oil traders.[49] The trade routes that went through the Promised Land were geographically the perfect place to connect the Middle East and North Africa. This is, in large part, how Solomon was able to later build a vast, wealthy empire. Genesis tell us that the caravan was on the way to Egypt, routing through the Promised Land with spices, balms, and myrrh.[50] Joseph was sold for 20 pieces of silver.

The irony that you already know, of course, is that the brothers who sold him later must appear before him after Joseph rises to become second in command over Egypt- where Potiphar, a high commanding officer, originally purchased him from the essential oil traders. When Joseph, who has not yet revealed himself to his brothers sends them back to his father Jacob with food (they came to him

---

[46] Numbers 16:30

[47] Numbers 16:46-50

[48] *Essential Oils Pocket Reference*, pp132-133.

[49] See *Healing Oils of the Bible*, xviii.

[50] See Genesis 37:25 and the surrounding story.

because of a famine that hit the entire world; Joseph was fore-warned by Pharaoh's dream and had Egypt prepare), the *greater irony* is this: he sends them with a gift of *the same essential oils* that the traders were carrying the very day he was sold!

Searching the Scripture, I also found that the incense in the temple was of a sweet smell.[51] History tells us that Romans cleansed public buildings, including temples, by diffusing essential oils. The oils could be steamed or burnt like incense- something you actually see in the Tabernacle that Moses built as well. The Romans, too, used aromatherapy in their baths to fight off disease and infection, as well as to invigorate themselves emotionally and physically.[52] **Essential oils weren't an isolated phenomena**.

We know that the wise men brought Jesus gifts of gold, frankincense, and myrrh. Two of these items are essential oils. Apparently, the ancients believed that frankincense had healing properties- it would be common in that culture for a healer or doctor to carry such an oil with him. The healing properties of frankincense are well documented even today.

When I was reviewing Jesus' birthday gifts from the magi, I came across the following quote: "Myrrh is still recognized for its ability to help with infections of the skin and throat and to regenerate skin tissue. Because of its effectiveness in

> There are hundreds of references in the Bible alone, meaning the authors must have assumed we would know what they were talking about.

preventing bacterial growth, myrrh was also used for embalming."[53] In other words, the author seems to point to the burial uses of myrrh as an after-thought, not as a primary use.

I always thought the wise men gave Jesus the gifts to signify His destiny:

- *Gold*- because He is a king

- *Frankincense*- because He is a healer

- *Myrrh*- to prepare Him for death and burial, because He is our sacrifice

---

[51] Exodus 30:25f.

[52] *Essential Oils Pocket Reference*, p5.

[53] *Essential Oils Pocket Reference*, p5.

Maybe so. But Jesus didn't need a long-term solution for body decay. In His sovereignty, the Father knew Jesus was a short-term grave sitter. *So why would Jesus need myrrh?*

Is it possible that Jesus used myrrh to heal the lepers? Given the fact that many traveling healers in the day would have had both frankincense and myrrh with them at all times, it seems plausible to think so.

Does this make the Bible stories less dramatic, less supernatural? *Not at all.*

As I was studying this information, I wondered why the Bible doesn't explain all of this to us. Here's what I came up with- see if it makes sense. The Bible doesn't explain everything. For instance, it doesn't even explain crucifixion- the very centerpiece of the entire book. The practice was so common that the authors just assume we'd "get it."

For example, If you read a news story on the Internet that said LeBron James did a windmill dunk on two defenders, you'd know exactly what that meant. You're probably envisioning it in your mind right now. I don't have to tell you what a windmill is, what a dunk is, or that they were even playing basketball. You've got it.

Why? Because those are common, everyday terms. No additional information needed.[54]

My guess is the same with essential oils. They were common. Everybody used them when they could. There are hundreds of references in the Bible alone, meaning the authors must have assumed we would know what they were talking about. We don't, though, without a bit of study- we understand them no more than people 2,000 years from now will know what a windmill dunk is without looking back at a few highlight films to get some clarification.

Of course, it's helpful to see that there are Egyptian hieroglyphics that date back to 5,000 years ago and *seem* to have renderings of essential oils. We know that Hippocrates, a famous Greek physician, used essential oils as his medicines. They were published in his works 400 years *before* the time of Christ. As Scott Johnson writes, "ancient texts and historical and archaeological evidence- including Egyptian hieroglyphics, Chinese manuscripts, Greek physicians'

---

[54] "The Bible contains 33 species and more than 500 references to essential oils and the aromatic plants from which they came" (Stewart, *Healing Oils of the Bible*, p7).

records, and Biblical references- suggest that **essential oils have been an integral part of health and wellness for centuries.**"[55]

And here's another interesting tidbit: "The word *doctor* only occurs three times in the Bible..."[56] In each instance, written by Luke (a physician, who would know what a *doctor* is), the reference is to "doctors of the law"- meaning *rabbis* or *teachers* as opposed to practitioners of healing.

In seminary, I learned about a rule of thumb called "the law of first mention." It means that in order to understand something, you look at when it first appears in the Bible and begin drawing your conclusions there. For instance, we know that people were created to walk and talk with God intimately, because that's how we first see people interacting with their Father in Genesis. A healthy relationship with God looks more like that that the rule-driven culture of Deuteronomy.

The first Biblical reference to a practitioner of healing is in the final chapter of Genesis. In Genesis 50:2, Joseph ordered the Egyptian physicians to embalm him. David Stewart makes a case that Jacob would have been embalmed in an Egyptian manner, then, effectively meaning that they used essential oils to embalm him.[57] Physicians, then, were those skilled in the use of essential oils.

> I was always told that any use of oils in the Bible was purely symbolic. *But was it really?* Or was it *symbolic* in the same way that I'd been taught about the wine Jesus created at the wedding feast being more like grape juice?

Go, lay hands on the sick and...

When Jesus sent His disciples to heal people, Mark adds an interesting factoid that the other Gospel writes don't cover: "They drove out many demons and anointed many sick people *with oil* and healed them."[58]

---

[55] *Surviving When Modern Medicine Fails*, p8. Emphasis added.

[56] See p49 of David Stewart's *Healing Oils of the Bible*. The references are Luke 2:46, Luke 5:17, Acts 5:34.

[57] See *Healing Oils of the Bible*, p49.

[58] Mark 6:13, New International Version. Emphasis mine.

My Dad is a Southern Baptist preacher. I went to church the Sunday after I was born. Then every Sunday morning, Sunday night, and Wednesday night after that. I was always told (the few times it ever even came up) that any use of oils in the Bible was purely symbolic. *But was it really?* Or was it *symbolic* in the same way that I'd been taught about the wine Jesus created at the wedding feast being more like grape juice? (It's ok to laugh.)

What if Jesus really did use essential oils at times and taught His disciples to do the same thing? In my mind, it doesn't make healing any less miraculous. He healed many with a word or command. And I believe, now, after having looked closer, that He likely healed others with a touch and applying essential oils.

Let me show you an instance in which we see Jesus with non-symbolic, totally legit, full-strength, essential oils. One would know the value of oils simply from reading the New Testament alone. When the "woman of the street" (probably Mary Magdalene) anointed Jesus' feet with oil, we know that Judas' objection was not the symbolism or imagery but the extravagant waste![59]

"It could have been sold for a year's wages and the money given to the poor!"[60]

Remember, too, that the vessel that contained the oil was an alabaster flask- the same type of container used in Egypt where Jesus and Moses presumably learned about the use of oils.[61]

James, Jesus' little brother, later wrote to his church that those who are sick should call the elders of the church to come lay hands on them, pray, and anoint them with oil.[62] What did James mean? Is it possible he learned about essential oils from his older brother?

After looking at the thrust of Scripture, it seems *extremely* unlikely to me that people in the Bible were just using symbolic oils with no medicinal qualities. In fact, I would say that *clearly* they are using oils that have healing power in them. Of course, the same God who was empowering them by His Spirit to lay hands

---

[59] The oil was spikenard, which, according to the *Essential Oils Pocket Reference*, is "used only by priests, kings, or high initiates." It was "one of the most precious oils in ancient times."

[60] Mark 14:5, New Living Translation. Presumably, she broken open an alabaster flask- the same material the Egyptians used to store oils.

[61] Matthew 26:7 draws out this detail.

[62] James 5:14

on the sick was also the same God who created and infused those plants with the oils in the first place.

Did Jesus travel throughout Galilee using His stock of frankincense and myrrh to cure the lame, cleanse the lepers, and cause the blind to see? When He sent His disciples out two by two- and then later sent out the 70- did He send them with some of that stock? **Are the magi more than just bit players in the nativity scene?** Were they the ones who gave Jesus the initial supply He needed to launch His healing ministry?

We don't know if He did things that way or not. Both ways- we don't know that He did, but we don't know that He did not either. In other words, it's possible.

Jesus didn't always heal instantly

Let me show you another fun tidbit that causes me to lean in the direction of "Jesus used essential oils" camp, though. There are several Greek words (the New Testament was originally written in Greek and Aramaic) for *healing*.[63] Here are two:

- *Iaomai*- means "miraculous" and "instantaneous" healing. This is how we often think Jesus healed, though this word only appears 30 times in the New Testament.[64]

- *Therapeuo*- means "to serve, to attend to, or to wait upon menially" and "to heal gradually over time with care."[65] This word appears 40 times in the Bible- a bit more than the instant cures we usually associate with miracles.

Here's what I'm getting at: we would say that *all* of Jesus' healings were miracles. None of us would make a list and say this one doesn't count, that one was normal, that one was something else...

> Sometimes, Jesus heals instantly. Other times, He teaches people how to be well.

---

[63] The discussion on the two Greek words comes from David Stewart's *Healing Oils of the Bible*. See p91.

[64] See examples in Matthew 8:13, Mark 5:29, Luke 8:47, John 12:40.

[65] Matthew 4:23-24, Mark 1:34, Mark 6:13, Luke 5:15, Acts 5:16, Acts 8:7, Revelation 22:2.

Yet, the word that is used in the Gospels clearly shows us that Jesus didn't always heal immediately. Sometimes, He administered a series of healings and other times He likely taught people to be well.

Here's the shocker: When Jesus sent the disciples out to heal, He used the *therapeuo* word.[66]

Two words used for healing

	Appears	Meaning	Happens
iaomai	30 times	Instantaneous healing	Spontaneously, in the moment
therapeuo	40 times	To serve, to attend to, or to wait upon menially- even by teaching them to be well	Intentionally, over time

I absolutely believe in instantaneous healing, *iaomai*. I've seen it firsthand.

- My brother gouged an eye when he was younger. He was never supposed to be able to see. Today, his eye is completely whole and has been for over 35 years. He doesn't even wear glasses. That's *iaomai*.

- My sister had a severe heart murmur when she was a small child. My parent's took her to a specialist in Houston who charted the arrhythmia. My Dad prayed and then took her back a few weeks later. The physician asked if they could use the new chart side-by-side in his classes with the old chart- one to show what a sick heart looked like on paper and the other to show what a perfect heart looked like. They still use that chart 30-plus years later. Again, that's *iaomai*.

- My uncle died twice at UAB. He came back. Twice. They didn't pump, aggressively resuscitate, or shock him. The doctor walked to the waiting room both times and said, "Another miracle." That was 15 years ago. Another *iaomai*.

So, yes, I believe Jesus heals people in the moment. I also believe He can do things in other ways, too. Specifically, I believe He can use natural means over

---

[66] See Matthew 10:8, for instance, as well as Luke 10:9 when Jesus sends the 70 out.

time in the same way that He also uses medical professionals. It's all His healing, anyway.

Matthew 8 reveals much about this healing spectrum. Specifically, the stories in this chapter tell us "how" Jesus heals people. We will look at each of these instances and make a few more observations about healing in general.

First, we know that Jesus *can* heal instantly. And that He *does*. In one of His first miracles, Jesus goes to Peter's house. There, we see Peter's mother-in-law is ill with a fever. Remarkably, Jesus touches her hand, the fever leaves her, and she serves them (8:15). He heals her in a moment. This is an example of *iaomai*. Just like my brother, my sister, and my uncle.

Second, we see that Jesus often teaches people to be well. Word gets out about Peter's mother-in-law (in the story above), and the townspeople began flocking to the house. Here's how it reads: "When evening came, many who were demon-possessed were brought to him, and He drove out the spirits with a word and healed all the sick."[67]

- Matthew 8:16 tells us that everyone in the town who is demon-possessed and sick is brought to Jesus. He heals *all* of them, according to the Bible (8:16).

- The phrase "with a word... healed all who were sick..." literally means, according to most Bible commentators that I've checked, "***He taught them to be well***" (8:16).

Want to guess what Greek word is used there in the New Testament? That's right, *therapeuo*, the other word for healing.

Sometimes, Jesus heals instantly. Other times, He teaches people how to be well. Make note, sometimes Jesus touches us and we are dramatically changed. Other times, He imparts His wisdom to us so that we can be changed. For example:

- Jesus can heal lung cancer- but *He can also teach us about the ills of smoking.*

- He can cure diabetes- *He also shows us how to eat better.*

---

[67] Matthew 8:16, New International Version.

- He can heal us of sexually transmitted diseases. Also, *He provides us with directions on how to live whole and healthy lives, as well as experience the joy of true intimacy.*

Why does He do this? I think many times it occurs because Jesus breaks the yoke of the original bondage, then *He teaches us how to walk in freedom.*

In John 5, we read the story of Jesus healing the man who sat paralyzed by the Pool of Bethesda. You probably know the story fairly well. He has been sick for 38 years.[68] As such, he has gathered in a place where many sick people gather. They all believed that whoever jumped into the pool first, when the waters stirred, would be healed.[69] He had likely seen people healed because he explained to Jesus that he had no one to push him in when the waters stir.

"Someone always jumps in ahead of me," he said, excusing his condition.[70]

Jesus asked if he actually wanted to be well. The man offered excuses as to why he could not be.[71] In spite of the man's reservations, Jesus healed the man.[72] Notice that He didn't lay hands on the man; He simply commanded him to gather his things and walk! That is clearly *iaomai.*

> Now… he must walk in health and wholeness or he can become sick again. In other words, *therapeuo* and *iaomai* are not opposed to each other- they always complement and enhance.

Here's an oddity: we later read that the man didn't even know it was Jesus that healed him, because he's not certain who Jesus even is! The man begins walking and is instantly bombarded by the religious leaders. They chide him for carrying his mat on the Sabbath.[73] A bit later, Jesus runs into the man (who,

---

[68] John 5:5

[69] John 5:3-4

[70] John 5:7

[71] John 5:6-7

[72] John 5:8. This to me goes against the argument that some people have about "not having enough faith." All throughout the New Testament Jesus heals people that have no faith. It doesn't seem, to me, to be a prerequisite.

[73] John 5:10

again, doesn't even know who Jesus is), telling him "go and sin no more, lest something worse happen to you" (worse than a 38-year illness!).[74]

Here's where I think the concept of *therapeuo* comes into play here: The man received an instant healing, an *iaomai*. Now, though, he must walk in health and wholeness or he can become sick again. In other words, **therapeuo and iaomai are not opposed to each other- they always complement and enhance.**

We see both types of healing in Paul's ministry, too.[75] After the shipwreck in Acts 27, Paul, Luke (who is writing Acts), and the others find themselves as the beneficiaries of Chief Publius' hospitality.

Luke writes, "Now in the neighborhood of that place were lands belonging to the chief man of the island, named Publius, who received us and entertained us hospitably for three days. It happened that the father of Publius lay sick with fever and dysentery. And Paul visited him and prayed, and putting his hands on him healed him. And when this had taken place, the rest of the people on the island who had diseases also came and were cured."[76]

Here's the kicker:

- The Bible tells us that Paul laid his hands on Publius' father and *iaomai* him- that is, he instantly healed him.

- The Bible tells us, too, that Paul *therapeuo* the rest of the island- and cured them.[77] That is, he "taught them to be well" and to continue walking in their healing.

Again, the Bible teaches both types of healing.[78]

---

[74] John 5:14

[75] I learned this example from *Healing Oils of the Bible*, p91.

[76] Acts 28:7-9, English Standard Version.

[77] I've seen instances where both words are translated as "cured" or "healed." So there is no direct correlation in the English language as to which Greek word is used here. Just know that the Bible teaches both types of healing.

[78] David Stewart writes, "Prayer can work without oils. Oils can work without prayer... If you are having success with prayer alone, it can be increased by the intelligent use of oils. If you are having success with oils, apply them with prayer and you will see even greater success" (*Healing Oils of the Bible*, p93).

I told you earlier than when Jesus sent the 12 out, He empowered them to *therapeuo*. This does not mean that they didn't *iaomai*, but it should encourage us from being discouraged when healing takes an extended time.

No doubt, you know people who were sick for years- and then were miraculously healed. Now they are walking in healing. In their example- perhaps it is your own- you see both types of healing working together.

In Luke 10, when Jesus sent the 70 out, He gave them instructions to *therapeuo* the sick- not *iaomai* them. Sure, *iaomai* can happen. But Jesus clearly told them to go teach people to be well. The same calling, I think, is available for all people today- to take healing with them wherever they go. **Many times we get to see *iaomai*; we always get to experience *therapeuo*.**

I started this chapter with a verse from Revelation 22:2. By now, you've guessed how this all fits together. "The leaves of the trees are for the *therapeuo* of the nations." Isn't that one of the places from which the oils are derived, from those leaves?

By the way, Paul says that *your life and the gifts you share with others* are a sacrifice and a fragrant offering to the Lord.[79] For some reason, I always linked this concept to the animal sacrifices of the Old Testament. I'm not so sure that makes the most sense, though, because Jesus completed all sacrificing on the Cross.

"It is finished," He said. No more sacrifice needed.

If you think about the aromas of the essential oils, though, and how intricately woven into the Tabernacle they were… into the place where sacrifices were made… perhaps this makes sense. It was the oils that brought peace and a sense of ease to the people. The aromas enlivened their senses and reminded them that God was near- and that He was for them. That is what you carry to everyone you see- it is what you do and who you are.[80]

---

[79] Philippians 4:18, Romans 12:1-2

[80] *Healing Oils of the Bible* says "Aromas of the essential oils used in the incenses, anointing oils, and sacrifices of worship among the Jews and early Christians" are a more likely reference here than the animals that were being slaughtered (see xvii in Stewart's book).

Why haven't I heard of this before?

Why don't we know about this stuff?

First, we've lost the information. History shows us that the oils made their way from the ancient civilizations all the way north to Europe, by the 1100s.

There's even a tale of a band of four thieves that worked during the bubonic plague of the 15th century. Roaming the streets of Marsaille, France, they allegedly robbed people who were dying of the plague- and even those who had died- without ever becoming infected themselves.

Once captured, the men revealed they had used a homemade blend of 50 cloves, rosemary, and other aromatic oils. They explained that they would rub their oil blend on their hands, ears, and temples. Soon thereafter, "the secret of the thieves was made public and the formula was posted in the city."[81]

> ... throughout the Dark Ages many libraries were burned. Knowledge was lost. Things were forgotten. Then other things were learned.

Of course, throughout the Dark Ages many libraries were burned. Knowledge was lost. Things were forgotten. Then *other* things were learned.

Now, second, we've created an environment in which we don't *need* to recover the lost information. Of course, I use the word *need* very loosely. My point is that we all have other options.

For instance, we don't need to find a remedy like Thieves for killing bacteria and infections, because we have over-the-counter drugs and prescriptions. They're five minutes away at the local pharmacy- no research and learning required.

My friend Gary (he and his wife were two of the people in the room at Gary's dining room that I told you about in the previous chapter) posted on FaceBook *tonight* that he's been taking the oils for 100 days, now. He's the guy that had the bad back and hiked around the Sandalwood farms and zip lined without a problem. His 100 days of oils have replaced 600 Advil and 300 Tylenol.[82] *Outstanding.*

---

81 Gary Young, *An Introduction to Young Living Essential Oils*, p4.

82 FaceBook wall post, 03-20-2014.

But before that he had learned to tolerate the pain, no matter how intolerable, with a heavy dose of pills. Who needs Valor when you can take Valium? And how many people are tolerating what my friend Gary once did before he (listened to his wife, like the other guys in the book, and) experienced true healing?

Third, you could argue that our medical establishment has a vested interest in keeping alternative remedies "out of sight" and "out of mind." And when they can't do that, they just try to discredit it- no matter how many positive results are out there.

I'm not knocking the establishment. If I break a bone, I'm going to the doctor. But you have to admit, something is amiss in our Western system of health. The U.S. spends more per capita on medical care than any other nation and consistently has worse results.[83]

The World Health Organization defines *health* as "a state of complete physical, mental and social well-being and not merely the absence of disease or infirmity." In the West, we seem content to focus on reactive solutions not proactive ones. In other words, we tend to treat rather than prevent. We look to eliminate sickness rather than walk in wholeness.

> In the West, we seem content to focus on reactive solutions not proactive ones. In other words, we tend to treat rather than prevent.

This seems to be true anywhere that medical solutions are sought *to the exclusion of* natural ones. Yes, there is always a place for medicine and doctors. I'm grateful for them. But a lifestyle that embraces walking in wholeness and healing (i.e., "Jesus taught them to be well") rather than fixing aches and pains seems best.

Those two choices are often financially at odds with one another. And, as you know, people do strange things for money. It divides family and friends, and it becomes the grid whereby all decisions are made.

When a medical condition is diagnosed as "chronic," we most often interpret the meaning as "There is no cure. It's terminal. We're stuck with this." However, a

---

[83] See http://www.americashealthrankings.org/Rankings/InternationalComparisons, for instance. Accessed 04-07-2014.

better response *might* be, "We don't yet know the cure. It might be out there- we just haven't discovered it, yet."[84]

David Stewart makes the case that "If we restrict ourselves to what the medical community has to offer, most of the time we will have cut ourselves off from any hope of real healing."[85] I don't know that I would say "most of the time," but I would agree that our options for health and wholeness will be *extremely limited.*

In *Surviving When Modern Medicine Fails,* Scott Johnson reminds us that medical options tend to shrink when technology becomes unavailable. He looks to Hurricane Katrina (2005), the Japanese Tsunami (2011), and other like natural disasters. During a 2005 tsunami in Indonesia, 45% of health clinics were "completely" or "seriously" damaged. Some islands lost all of their X-ray and generator equipment. Scott doesn't try to paint a "doom and gloom" scenario- just point to our dependence on technologies that may not always be available.[86]

> ... a lifestyle that embraces walking in wholeness and healing (i.e., "Jesus taught them to be well") rather than fixing aches and pains seems best.

A few months ago, my home city of Birmingham shut down for a few days. It happened abruptly when a mix of snow and ice formed. Cars were stopped on the highways by the hundreds. People found themselves sleeping in shopping malls and offices while their kids were stranded for days at their schools. No one died, but access to medical technology was virtually halted. Natural remedies know no such boundaries, however.

During my research for this book I read parts of the *Essential Oils Pocket Reference.* That book sums up a future possibility quite well:

> *Our modern world has only begun the discovery of the power of God's healing oils- something the ancient world knew well... The earth and its healing oils were the ancient world's medicine- something our modern world should take note of and embrace."* The guide concludes that "the

---

[84] *Healing Oils of the Bible*, p14.

[85] *Healing Oils of the Bible*, p14.

[86] *Surviving When Modern Medicine Fails*, pp16-17

way to live with strength and vitality without pain and disease lies in what God has created, not in what man has altered.[87]

I like this phrase, especially: "These oils are God's medicines." Then- "When we put the oils on, we don't first feel a medical change, rather, we feel a spiritual shift... something is changing..." In light of where they came from... and the history of how Jesus and the disciples and the early church used them, doesn't that make sense that the Spirit would shift first and then the body would come in alignment...?

"God gave us these oils to live in Heaven while hell is all around us," said Gary.

Healing Oils of the Bible reminds us that the oils are creations of God's actual words.[88] That's true. Re-read Genesis 1. The plants are not stained by sin, feelings of guilt & shame, or relational distrust. This is, perhaps, why Gary said to the Frenchman that "essential oils are as close to God as we can get."

> ...the oils are creations of God's actual words.

God gave this to you... in the beginning

By the way, Genesis 1:29-30 tells us that God gave us every plant and tree for "food." The actual Hebrew word that is used is *oklah*.[89] God gave every plant and tree for *oklah*. The word *oklah* includes things you eat, but it is more- it includes medicines.[90] In other words, **there were medicines in the first plants- even before sin.**

I wondered about this: *Why would God provide medicines in the beginning, before sin and sickness entered the human condition?*

If you go back to the differences between *iaomai* and *therapeuo*, though, the answer becomes clearer. Quite simply, God's intent was- and remains- for

---

[87] *Essential Oils Pocket Reference*, p9.

[88] *Healing Oils of the Bible*, p17.

[89] The New Testament was originally penned in Greek and Aramaic; the Old Testament was originally written in Hebrew.

[90] See *Healing Oils of the Bible*, xix.

people to walk in wholeness and healing. He was going to "teach them to be well," I believe.

The implications are astounding if you go back to that "law of first mention" concept I discussed a few pages back. Grasp it: **the first time God gives Adam stewardship of the plants He is giving Adam food and healing**.

That's good. Really good. And that's the way it was from the beginning. Let's embrace new technologies and not overlook anything that might be helpful for us. At the same time, let's not forget the oldest and purest solutions of all.

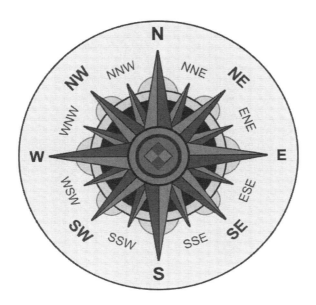

02: Direction: re-read your history

Action steps

☐ Reach out to someone in your upline- a guy. There aren't a lot of guys that are enrolled as distributors, so

The main idea: Let's embrace new technologies and not overlook anything that might be helpful for us. At the same time, let's not forget the oldest and purest solutions of all.

you're probably going to have to get your wife to help you on this one... get her to reach out to a woman who has a husband who is supportive of her business. Go grab dinner with them and listen to his story. The odds are that he was extremely skeptical at first- maybe even for awhile. If his wife his having significant success in Young Living, that has likely changed. Learn what you can.

☐ Join a FaceBook guys group. If you're in our line, I can invite you into ours. If you're not, I'll help you connect with some guys that have one where you are. Guys post on our wall just about every single day. Sometimes it's nonsensical, sometimes it's impressively deep and wise. It's always encouraging. Plus, now I have some friends who are on the same journey- some I've met face-to-face and some that I will at some point in the future.[91] The stuff shared on the wall in this group is way different than what's share on the "open group" that is comprised 98% of some great women. If you've been to that wall, you know what I mean.

Want to know more?

☐ Read:

    ☐ "Aromatherapy: An Ancient Science Returns to the Modern World," Chapter 1 in *Aromatherapy: The Essential Beginning*, by D. Gary Young

    ☐ "Yesterday's Wisdom, Tomorrow's Destiny," Chapter 1 in *Essential Oils Pocket Reference*, Life Science Publishing

    ☐ "God: The First Aromatherapist," Chapter 1 in *Healing Oils of the Bible*, David Stewart.

☐ Listen:

    ☐ To the relevant chapter of the audiobook

☐ Search:

    ☐ Review the World Health Organization website briefly (http://www.who.int/en/) See what trends you can discover about health in the U.S. in particular- compared to other developed countries around the world. Is a lifestyle of *therapeuo* a solution for some of our ails?

---

[91] You're reading the stories of some of these guys throughout this book.

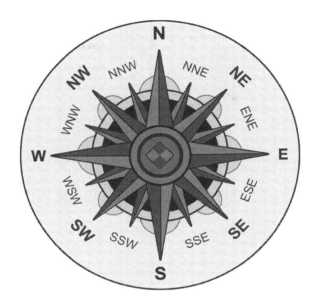

02: A diffuser is a what? / Verick's story

So, my wife brings this thing she calls a "diffuser" home from a friend's house. I asked her the obvious questions: "What are you going to diffuse?"

It seemed like she was going new age on me, but she explained that there was this stuff called Thieves oil that would kill the mold in our rental house. I was for that, because who likes mold?

Verick Burchfield's wife, Crystal, has been involved with Young Living since 2011. They've been married for 16 years and have four kids.

Fast forward about a year and she has been diffusing Thieves the whole time and the house smells great. We then move to another location and she actually starts using other Young Living essential oils in the diffuser and then on herself!

This is where I started getting a little weirded out. I am a Nurse Practitioner and work in an ER, so when she started talking about using oils on herself for health and thinking about using them on our kids, I just shut her down. There was no way she was going to use that voodoo on us. We actually called her The Shaman...

She did what she knew to do. She prayed about it and felt led to continue using oils in spite of my resistance to them. She also began researching their reported use for different ailments and studied about asthma. My youngest son has had asthma since he was very little. He had RSV at a very young age and we were told that he would always have respiratory problems. This translated into almost 3-4 hospitalizations yearly, in spite of daily use of 4 adult dose asthma medicines.

My wife had experienced severe health problems and had been miraculously healed of them. She felt impressed to begin using the oils on him for his asthma. We started to see improvement in his symptoms immediately. At his next asthma doctor visit, his peak flow numbers were improved from the previous one. My wife shared with the doctor what she was doing. The doctor, pleased with the results, actually agreed that we could begin to decrease my son's medicines slowly.

I watched in amazement over a 6 month period— my son came off every single medicine he took for asthma. Instead, he was now on a daily topical application of Breathe Again, Valor, and R.C., with Dorado Azul for any breakthroughs. I couldn't argue with what I was seeing. I was convinced then and there. Late last Spring, my 8 year old ran his first 5k race with me. We won overall. This further sealed the fact in my head that these oils could be very helpful.

Simultaneously, I started watching the size of my wife's oils order increasing. This meant more money was coming out of our budget. I was nervous, but we were getting such good results and the general health of the house was improving. Nonetheless, the money issue was a bone of contention.

But then she started sharing her story with others. They started "signing up" under her and she began teaching classes. At this point, she was doing a home business about oils. I was fine with it, because each month it would help offset the cost of the oils.

She felt the Lord called her to share, because of how much it had helped us. It was a ministry in her eyes, and it was growing. Within 6 months she was paying for her own oils and trying to juggle this growing business. Like many others guys' wives she was handling it with grace. Quickly, her "small" home business was beginning to explode. She was teaching classes multiple times a week and even began asking me to be a part every now and then.

It wasn't long before I was using the oils on myself. I am a running fanatic. I love it, and even though I'm in my late thirties I am still trying to increase my personal best times. She suggested En-R-Gee for exercise and Motivation for mental focus while I'm at work. I decided to combine the two, and I soon noticed that when I applied them before a run, I consistently ran about 90 seconds faster per 4 miles than when I didn't use them. To me that was life altering. I began using it every time I ran, and there was virtually no fatigue. So once again, I was sold on the oils.

In the Fall of 2013, I was completely in my wife's corner regarding her oils business. So much so, that I started taking over some of her responsibilities in the home. Namely homeschooling. The "hobby" of oils had quickly grown into a business that was helping our family out health-wise and financially! More than I could have imagined, back when she first started diffusing Thieves.

Now, I have gone from complete skeptic, to an amazed dad, to a happy semi-athlete, to a proud husband, and- the last stage- a coworker with my wife. I am now studying the oils daily and helping sign-up people with my wife. We have a common goal and vision for our next steps in both Young Living and in life. I am working with the woman I love, who was patient through the times of my doubt and arguing. She was patient when I didn't know anything about oils and has taught me more than I could imagine.

If I could offer any advice to guys reading this, it would be to believe in your wife. Help her any way you can, and respect what she is doing. You will not only learn something, you will also be helping others and- most of all- growing your marriage.

_ Verick Burchfield, Crystal's husband

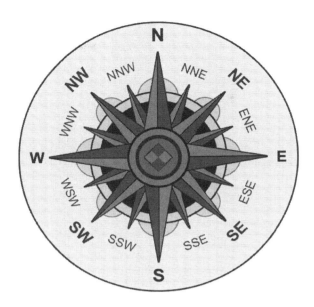

03: Essential oils 101

Proverbs 21:20 tells us that *"There is* treasure to be desired and oil in the dwelling of the wise."[92]

If your wife has had her oils for any length of time at all, you've probably seen enough evidence to know the truth of this verse firsthand. By now, you've probably seen her knock out enough fevers, mend countless cuts and bruises, and soothe enough sleepless nights that you wonder

> **Main idea:** Essential oils are a small, unique part of each plant. They are, in a sense, part of the life force of that plant, each plant having a unique version of its own.

what you were doing before the oil kit arrived. In fact, I find myself astonished at the number of nuisances we used to simply tolerate- things like snoring, warts, chest congestion, sleepless nights for the kids…

Aside from the financial gain we've experienced as distributors of the oils, I've seen the truth of Proverbs 21:20 firsthand. The oils have changed how we do life.

---

[92] King James Version.

Let me give you some background on the verse. Solomon, the author of Proverbs, is the richest, wisest man that ever lived. Some economists estimate that if Solomon's wealth was calculated into current dollars, he would be a *trillionaire*. That net worth is more than anybody on earth. In fact, you could probably add the top two guys together and Solomon would still surpass them combined.[93]

Tradition, as well as the the Bible, says that people traveled from all over the world just to listen to him talk. And when they did, they would stand amazed at his wisdom. Even with the little things like how his servants entered and exited the palace and how he conducted basic, everyday affairs the guests were always impressed. They were spellbound, captivated by his knowledge and attention to every detail.[94] The way he led his kingdom left them speechless, *because it all made so much sense.*[95]

At the beginning of Solomon's reign, the Lord actually asked him what he'd like. Many scholars say that Solomon wouldn't have been more than 18-21 years at the time, meaning he was given every high school and frat boy's dream: a guaranteed "your wish is my command" scenario from the Creator. In a word, Solomon asked for this: *wisdom*. And because of his request for wisdom (and not the things that would have been at the *top* of my list), the Lord responded in an amazing way:

> Since this is your heart's desire and you have not asked for wealth, possessions or honor, nor for the death of your enemies, and since you have not asked for a long life but for wisdom and knowledge to govern my people over whom I have made you king, therefore wisdom and knowledge will be given you. And I will also give you wealth, possessions and honor, such as no king who was before you ever had and none after you will have.[96]

In the other words, Solomon asked for the most important thing, and ended up getting *everything else* with it.

So, what does this have to do with essential oils? Well, as I contemplated how my wife began her journey into natural remedies and essential oils, I remember

---

[93] http://www.forbes.com/billionaires/ accessed 03-24-2014.

[94] His story is found in 1 Kings 1-11.

[95] 1 Kings 10:1-13 details how this happened to the Queen of Sheba.

[96] 2 Chronicles 1:11-12, New International Version.

her strong desire to gain wisdom and knowledge for the sole purpose of taking care of her family. She wanted to protect our children from illness and be able to comfort/treat them when illness came knocking.

Her request before the Lord was, "I want to manage what you've trusted me with in a wise and educated manner." He has certainly answered her request with a resounding, "I will give you wisdom and even more…!" And that's where we come in, fellow comrades. When it comes to taking care of our families, we as husbands have the unique privilege of partnering with the wisdom our wives have already tapped into regarding essential oils. The Lord is eager to "give it all" to you.

- **Take that Proverb to heart**- and realize that oils are found in the homes of the wise. And, no, Solomon wasn't talking about olive oil or motor oil.[97]

- **Learn about the oils.** That is, the oils won't do much good stashed away in the fancy carrier that your wife bought or resting in your medicine cabinet.

- **Study the compensation plan.** This is how your wife will get paid. I'll share a story with you in a future chapter about how one pastor took this head-on and saw his wife's business explode from one month to the next.[98]

- **Get behind your wife's efforts to grow her business.** She'll likely be more successful with you on board than she will on her own. If she's succeeding right now, like my wife was, think about how much *greater* she'll be with you helping her!

What are essential oils?

You probably have oils in your house right now- things like vegetable oil, peanut oil, and olive oil. These oils are great for cooking and even eating. Some of these household oils can even keep lanterns burning when the power goes out.

---

[97] I hope we established this in the previous chapter!

[98] I originally began penning this manuscript with a section about the compensation plan. It began occupying a disproportional amount of space in its chapter, so I put it in the appendix. Then the appendix was making this book too long, so look for a companion book to this one to release soon- *The Husband's Field Guide to the Comp Plan*.

These types of oils are considered "fatty" oils. If you rub cooking oil on your body, it will clog your pores. It doesn't mean that it's a *bad* oil, it just means that is not its proper use- any more than the screen door was made for a submarine, as the old joke goes.

Essential oils are different than those oils. They are aromatic, volatile liquids. They are often called *therapeutic* or *aromatic* oils. By the way, I hope you're making the connection between *therapeuo*, the word for healing that we studied in the previous chapter. If not, consider this your fair warning to circle the word, highlight it, or make a note in the margin of the book.

...as I contemplated how my wife began her journey into natural remedies and essential oils, I remember her strong desire to gain wisdom and knowledge for the sole purpose of taking care of her family.

Here's the non-scientific (read: *my*) version of what these essential / therapeutic / aromatic oils are:

> *Essentials oils are a small, unique part of each plant. They are in a sense part of the life force of that plant, each plant having a unique version of its own.*

It may not be scientifically thorough, but it helps me understand what they are, and where they come from, as well as, why different oils do different things. Now, here's something that somebody smarter than me wrote: "Essential oils are volatile liquids and aromatic compounds found within the shrubs, flowers, trees, roots, bushes, and seeds that are usually extracted through steam distillation."[99]

Pretty much what I said. Well, *kinda*.

Three characteristics of essential oils

I don't have time in this book to give you a list of various oils and what they do. There are plenty of books written on that already. Rather, I'd like to provide you with an overview of what the oils are and how they work. Consider this the equivalent of "Mechanic Shop 101"- or "Oils for Dummies."

---

[99] *Essential Oils Pocket Reference*, p15. A similar quote appears on p1 of the reference guide, as well.

The first thing you need to know is essential oils are *concentrated*- so they are far more potent than dried herbs.

Now, it takes a large volume of plant material to produce a small quantity of oil. Get these examples:

- 5,000 pounds of rose petals result in 1 kilo of rose oil.[100] I had no idea what a kilo of oil equated to, so I did a quick Google search. Turns out, a kilo is about a liter.

- For every 2,000 pounds of grapefruit you distill, you'll net about 1.5 pounds of essential oil.[101]

- It takes 2-3 tons of Melissa plant material to produce just one pound of Melissa oil.[102]

Yes, it takes a lot of plant material to make a drop of oil, but a small drop of oil then contains the full force of the entire plant- *of all of those plants*. When you have a bottle of rose oil, you have the life force of 5,000 pounds of roses. That's a lot of plant. And that means a lot of life.

Essential Oils are *extremely* concentrated chemical compounds that pack a powerful punch. Maybe this story will help explain it a bit. My kids like to go to the office with me. So, at least one of them rolls with me once every week or so. It's the advantage of having a job where I'm the boss and having kids that also homeschool.

> ... it takes a lot of plant material to make a drop of oil, but a small drop of oil then contains the full force of the entire plant- *of all of those plants*.

The guys at The Village are incredible with the kids. Since I have an "If you go to work, then you have to work" policy for my kids, that means that they have to actually *do something productive* when they go. No loafing around all day. This means my boys usually find themselves helping in the commercial kitchen where we have three meals going out a day for all the residents, or they end up sorting items at the thrift store, or renovating whatever project is being completed somewhere on-site.

---

[100] *Essential Oils Pocket Reference*, p1.

[101] "Core Vigor and Vitality" (in *School of Nature's Remedies* series), p3.

[102] *Essential Oils Desk Reference*, Fifth Edition, location 1.46.

The up-side is that they learn to work. The down-side is that they pick up the habits of some of the guys they work with.

Now, the guys at The Village have a certain drink they make- it's called a "sham." It comes straight from the prison halls, which should be a warning as to what I'm about to tell you. You mix a flavored soda (like Strawberry or Peach Fanta) *with* an energy drink *with* a small package of Kool-Aid. You mix it together, stir it up, and pour over ice. It's supposed to keep you awake, and (as you might imagine) it's rather successful.

One night after teaching a class, the guys made me one. I tried it, didn't like it, and was then encouraged that it was "an acquired taste." *Perhaps, but no thanks.*

Well, the men were making shams one day and thought my boys might like to get in on the action. They were wise enough not to give the boys a soda without my permission (I probably would have given it; just being honest), and had enough sense not to offer them a Monster energy drink. But they gave them each a packet of Kool-Aid. When I picked-up the boys from the kitchen, their faces were stained with red and orange. And they were all *hyper, hyper, hyper!*

"We made some Kool-aid," Mr. Charles told me.

After some investigative work, I found out that they had been making Kool-aid on their own by pouring an entire packet into small, 10 ounce styrofoam cups. Those packages are designed to make up to a gallon of juice- 128 ounces! My kids were chugging it at almost 13 times the recommended dosage. Hence, the stains and the increased adrenalin levels. There is a *lot* packed into that one small packet of Kool-aid.

The same idea is true of essential oils. **They're like the concentrated Kool-aid of the natural healing world. Only they pack amazing, powerful molecular compounds of goodness.** A little bit of oil contains the power of *large* quantities of the plant, which is why you often dilute them. In comparison to their herbal counterparts, (herbs are dried/dehydrated plant matter) "essential oils are 100 to 10,000 times more concentrated than herb."[103]

In a moment, after looking at two more preliminary facts you need to know about essential oils, we'll tie all of the pieces together and I'll show you what this concentration-thing means and why it's a good thing (well, unless you're using Kool-aid).

---

[103] "Core Vigor and Vitality" (in *School of Nature's Remedies* series), p3.

The second thing you should understand is that they are small- I'm not talking atomic particle small, but we're talking small enough to slip and slide in and out of cells. Most essential oils have an extremely high oxygen content, which is another of the reasons they are so effective. The *Essential Oil Pocket Reference* says that "Essential oils have a unique ability to penetrate cell membranes and diffuse throughout the blood and tissues…" They can do that, in part, because they're tiny.

The third thing to remember is that they travel. Yep, they move. Let me give it to you in official language and then I'll give you an illustration.

Here's what Gary writes: "When applied to the body by rubbing on the feet, essential oils will travel throughout the body and affect every cell, including the hair, within 20 minutes."[104]

If you apply an essential oil topically (that means you put it on your skin):

- Within 20-30 seconds, the oil enters your blood stream.

- Within 20-30 minutes, it has circulated throughout your body.

- Within 2-3 hours, your body has sufficiently metabolized it.

By the way, you can apply them topically, you can inhale them (put the bottle to your nose and sniff or put a drop on your hands and cup your hands around your face to create your own personal nirvana-

> A little bit of oil contains the power of *large* quantities of the plant, which is why you often dilute them.

moment), you can diffuse them (which is a less direct method of inhalation), and you can ingest Young Living oils (drink or swallow them after putting them in a capsule). *Please*, don't ingest a random essential oil from your local health food store or amazon.com. In fact, I wouldn't put it in my body if it doesn't meet the same standards that Young Living has set- and we haven't found another company with those standards. But more on that later.

Back to concentration… Scott Johnson taught an all-day class called "Nature's Remedies" in downtown Birmingham back in March.[105] According to Scott's own testimony (and pictures on the projector), he's lost about 50 pounds in his quest to become healthier and to live a continued lifestyle of wholeness. (He is a

---

[104] *Aromatherapy*, Gary Young, p21.

[105] Scott Johnson, opening session, Nature's Remedies conference, March 22, 2014. BJCC.

great example of Chapter 2, where I explained the difference between *iaomai* and *therapeuo*). Scott is living a lifestyle of *therapeuo*- and teaching others to do the same.)[106]

"The oils travel," he said. Then he described how lavender is a good oil to use if you have red eyes. He flashed a PowerPoint slide to illustrate his point and hit us with the whammy: "You can't use lavender directly in your eyes, though, or it will irritate them even more." Then, "In fact, you wouldn't want to put any essential oil directly into your eyes."

Remember, the oils are concentrated. Think 5,000 pounds of roses going into one bottle. Think one drop of those 5,000 roses going straight into your eyeball.

"So here's what you can do…" He placed some lavender on his fingers, just a few drops. "Run the lavender under your eyes. Like those football players do with the eye-black, to keep the light and the glare out of their eyes…"

I envisioned Tebow wearing purple flowers streaked across his face instead of "John 3:16" or "Ephesians 2:8."

Scott said you probably don't want to rub the lavender near your eyebrows, because the oils might drop into your eye. "You can also just put the drops on your palms and inhale."

His point was easy to takeaway: **the oils will move from your nasal cavity or from your cheekbones through your bodily system and hit the eyes internally within just a few moments.** Problem solved.

Here's the scientific mumbo-jumbo (and I use that term in the most polite, respectful way possible): "When a fragrance is inhaled, the odor molecules travel up the nose where they are trapped by olfactory membranes… the lining of the nose… When stimulated by odor molecules, this lining of nerve cells triggers electrical impulses to the olfactory bulb in the brain."[107] The impulses are transmitted throughout the limbic system of the brain, throughout areas where taste, emotions, and even memories are handled. The limbic system is

---

[106] The Young Living website says that "As Young Living's director of global education and U.S. sales, Scott draws upon his wealth of experience and diverse educational background to create and oversee the company's global training initiatives. His passion lies in bringing the secrets of natural healing to those who seek greater wellness." Go to http://www.youngliving.com/en_US/company/media/events/natures-remedies/presenters, accessed 03-30-2014.

[107] *Essential Oils Pocket Reference*, p25.

intertwined with the areas of the brain that control everything from your breathing to your heart rate to your stress load to your (or your wife's) libido![108]

Pretty amazing, huh? Ok, to sum up. Essential oils are:

- *Concentrated* (meaning "strong")
- *Small* (meaning, they can go into tiny places)
- *Travelers* (put it anywhere on or in your body and it effects all of you)

Three things essential oils are really good at

Now that you understand a little bit about what they're like, let me tell you some of the things they do. To keep it simple, I'll give you three. Again, you and I aren't chemists; we're normal, everyday guys who just want to walk in *therapeuo* and wholeness.

Remember, the oils run through your body… they're little concentrated-strength travelers. As they go, they interact with the living data (your cells) that are there. The oils have compounds in them. The compounds do three different things:

> … the oils run through your body… they're little concentrated-strength travelers. As they go, they interact with the living data (your cells) that are there.

First, they clean-up bad receptor sites. Your cells are constantly communicating with each other and with other parts of your body. But sometimes their ability to communicate gets jammed- like bad cell phone reception. When this happens, certain compounds in the oils jump in to clear the haze and get the signals restored.[109]

Second, they deprogram bad info. Here's the deal: your cells are duplicating themselves every day- some of them multiple times a day. If they get "bad code" in them, they're going to replicate the wrong way.

---

[108] I'll come back to this in chapter 5.

[109] These compounds are called phenols and phenylpropanoids. See *Healing Oils of the Bible*, by David Stewart, pp28-31.

Think of it like this: Michael Keaton played in the movie *Multiplicity* almost 20 years ago.[110] At some point, he decided he could get more work done if he duplicated or cloned himself. So he did. It worked so well that he made more copies of himself. But then the copies of himself started making their own copies- and those copies of copies of copies just got weirder and weirder and weirder.

It's kinda like that game you played when you were growing up, where one person tells another person a secret... they tell the next person... it goes around the room through ten or twenty more people... and sounds *nothing* like the original secret! That's what bad cells do.[111] Thankfully, there are compounds in the essential oils that make sure your cells are making good copies.[112]

Third, they reprogram with good info. It's not enough to simply clear up the communication lines, and then stop the bad communication. You've got to get good info traveling through the lines. That's where the reprogramming compounds come into play.[113]

Now, the compounds I referenced above appear in various oils at varying levels. This is why some are better at certain things than others. At the same time, it's why it can be ok to use *any essential* oil for a given situation, even if you don't have the specific one you need on hand. Because they can alter your body's structure at the cellular level, essential oils have the ability to re-write the DNA and alter cellular functioning, systematically repairing cells as they work through the body.[114]

Have you ever gotten a computer virus? I used to get them *all the time*, it seemed, when I was running a PC. I don't think I've ever gotten one in the 5 or 6 years that I've been running a Mac, but I still remember them. You could open a little email attachment- a "Trojan horse" picture or something. The virus would run through the entire system, rewriting the code for every bit of data you had in the computer. Eventually, the thing would become so weighted that it would crash.

---

[110] http://en.wikipedia.org/wiki/Multiplicity_(film), accessed 03-31-2014.

[111] For an interesting project, research "cancer and replication."

[112] These compounds are called sesquiterpenes. See *Healing Oils of the Bible*, by David Stewart, pp28-31.

[113] Monoterpenes. See *Healing Oils of the Bible*, by David Stewart, pp28-31.

[114] *Healing Oils of the Bible*, p28.

Essential oils are like that- except in reverse. They travel through the entire body, opening receptors, pushing out bad data and rewriting code to heal DNA. They bring health and vitality.

Let me give you a stat that will blow your mind. *Healing Oils of the Bible* suggests that each drop of essential oil contains 40 million-trillion molecules. That's a 4 with 19 zeros after it. It looks like this:

40,000,000,000,000,000,000

The author of the book, David Stewart compares the composition of our bodies, stating that "we have 100 trillion cells... a lot." When you look at how many molecules are in each drop- that's right, a single drop- of essential oils, you get a better perspective. Stewart continues that "one drop of oil contains enough molecules to cover every cell in our body with 40,000 molecules."[115]

When you remember that it only takes *one drop* in the right place at the right time for the right cell to communicate with the rest of your body, you can see just how profound the effects of a pure oil can be.

"...one drop of oil contains enough molecules to cover every cell in our body with 40,000 molecules."

You might need to recharge, like your phone

Everything has a frequency. Everything. Everything, well, except dead things, that is. Frequency is defined as "the measurable rate of electrical energy flow that is constant between any two points."[116]

Now, don't get confused with the type of electrical frequency that runs your appliances at home. Most of them run on an A.C. (alternating current) frequency of about 60 hertz. They are things made by man. Things made by God (people, plants, animals) operate with D.C. (direct current) frequency.[117]

---

[115] David Stewart, *Healing Oils of the Bible*, pp27-28.

[116] Gary Young, *Aromatherapy*, p35.

[117] Gary Young, *Aromatherapy*, p36.

A healthy human has a standing frequency of 62-68 MHz. As your state of health drops, so does that frequency. Your frequency is a measure of how strong and "alive" you really are.[118]

Consider what happens as your frequency descends:

- Cold symptoms manifest around 58 MHz, as at this point your immune system begins shutting down.[119]

- Flu symptoms surface around 57 MHz.

- Candida appears around 55 MHz.

- Cancer *can* begin when the body falls below 42 MHz.

- The process of dying begins about 25 MHz and bottoms at at 0 MHz when you are pronounced dead.

Royal Raymond Rife, a medical doctor who studied human frequencies in the early 1900s, discovered that he could actually *destroy* viruses and cancer cells at certain frequencies. He found that other frequencies prevented the development of disease.[120]

What does this have to do with essential oils? Well, here's the kicker, straight from Mr. Essential Oil himself: "Clinical research shows that essential oils have the highest frequency of any natural substance known to man, creating an environment in which disease, bacteria, virus, fungus, etc., *cannot* live."[121] Notice, those things *cannot* live. Not, "they prefer something else... so they can't thrive" but they *cannot even exist.*

I wondered just how high the frequency of essential oils might be, so I did a bit of reading. The numbers were astounding. The chart below will give you the details.[122] You'll see that the frequency of rose is about *five times* the frequency of a healthy human. Peppermint, a very commonly used oil (it's relatively

---

[118] This list comes from *Healing Oils of the Bible*, p32. See also Gary Young, *Aromatherapy*, p38.

[119] Gary Young, *Aromatherapy*, p38.

[120] Gary Young, *Aromatherapy*, p35.

[121] Gary Young, *Aromatherapy*, p40.

[122] This information comes from *Healing Oils of the Bible*, p33.

inexpensive and easy to get) is a full 10 MHz *higher* than a healthy reading. No wonder it gets people jazzed up!

Frequencies of selected essential oils

Essential oil	Frequency / MHz
Rose	320 MHz
Helichrysum	181 MHz
Lavender	118 MHz
Blue Tansy	105 MHz
German Chamomile	105 MHz
Juniper	98 MHz
Peppermint	78 MHz
Basil	52 MHz

The frequency of the oils is one of the reasons that the pain "goes away" almost immediately in many cases within a few minutes of applying certain oils.[123] Quite simply, a lower personal frequency means you are not feeling well- and all the symptoms of not feeling well (like pain) come with that. "One of the most important healing modalities of the oils is their ability to lift our bodily frequencies to levels where disease cannot exist."[124] Since an essential oil can raise your frequency, though, you start feeling better as your frequency elevates.

This is one of the chief reasons why Young Living's claim, that people who use essential oils have a 60% greater resistance to illness, may be true. And why YL argues that people who use essential oils recover 70% faster from any illnesses that they do contract.[125] Yes, you could contend that people who use essential oils tend to be more health conscious in the first place, and therefore would contract less illnesses anyway. Such is a circular argument, though, for a lifestyle of wholeness and healing is what we are seeking. The oils are a component of that.

---

[123] Gary Young, *Aromatherapy*, pp36-37.

[124] *Healing Oils of the Bible*, p33.

[125] Gary Young, *Aromatherapy*, p39.

On a side note, foods have frequencies, too. As you might suppose, a healthier food has a higher frequency. David Stewart writes, "fresh herbs measure 20-27 MHz... fresh produce 5-10 MHz. Processed or canned food measured *zero*. In other words, there is no life or life force in canned or processed foods."[126]

Now you have a scientific answer (another one) when your kids ask you why you don't like McDonald's. And you know why you feel like junk when you eat too much pizza. After learning about frequencies it's not hard to believe the old but true adage, "You are what you eat."

I wondered why Young Living never has coffee at their events. Ever. I approached more than one urn at the Hawaii event (with a coffee mug that was provided), only to find that I was filling my *coffee cup* with water!

I asked one of the execs, a lady, who politely told me, "*They* frown on it."

That *They* she used in her sentence led me to believe she, too, was a drinker, so I asked, "Do you drink?"

She quietly confirmed she did, and smiled shyly about the whole thing.

"I won't tell," I promised.

I should have added- "It's not like I'm going to go put it in a book or anything!"

Here's the scoop about coffee: simply holding a cup of coffee in your hand drops your body frequency by about 8 MHz. Take a sip and you're down by 6 more MHz.[127] Yes, essential oils can boost this right back up, but the YL stance on it seems to be, "Why would you mess with that in the first place?"

By the way, studies have shown that **your thoughts can raise and lower your frequencies**, too- by as much as 10 MHz in either direction![128] In other words, a bunch of negative guys sitting around drinking coffee makes for a bad day! So much for my plans of being a grumpy old guy who gets the free "senior coffee" at the local fast food restaurant, chomps down on a processed biscuit, reads the paper, and complains about how things used to be.

---

[126] *Healing Oils of the Bible*, p32. Emphasis added.

[127] *Healing Oils of the Bible*, p32.

[128] *Healing Oils of the Bible*, p33.

This is, in some sense, what the Bible may mean when Solomon (the guy who said wise people have oils in their house) says, "As a man thinks, so is he…"[129]

And get this: prayer makes an even greater change, notching someone's frequency up by 15 MHz![130] This means that a perfect scenario for bringing healing in your household, I believe, is the following:

- Walk in a lifestyle of health and healing (diet and exercise)

- Use the oils when they are needed

- Speak a positive confession as to what is going to happen

- Pray and thank God, declaring it to be true on earth as it is in Heaven

Understand, **your natural state is health and wholeness. Your body, when healthy is fighting for health**- not fighting for disease. Your body, when healthy and whole, is moving *higher* in frequency. On a Biblical level, this is because you

> "One of the most important healing modalities of the oils is their ability to lift our bodily frequencies to levels where disease cannot exist."

are created in God's image.[131] He *does not* have disease or illness.[132] And, there is no illness or sickness in Heaven. Jesus says that you live the presence of the Kingdom, now.[133] As such, healing, your naturally-created state as well as your end destination, are available in this present moment.

The oils simply "restore the body back to its natural state of balance and health at the most basic and fundamental levels." They may do this instantly (*iaomai*, as we learned in the previous chapter), over time (*therapeuo*), or a combination of both.[134] Again, healing is your natural state; you are naturally getting better not naturally getting worse.

---

[129] Proverbs 23:7

[130] *Healing Oils of the Bible*, p33.

[131] Genesis 1:27

[132] Some people believe God gives illness and sickness and disease to people. I do not believe this to be the case.

[133] Luke 12:32 and Luke 17:21, for instance.

[134] *Healing Oils of the Bible*, p31.

All men are created equal, but not all oils

We had the privilege to ride on the bus with Scott Johnson, Young Living's director of global education and U.S. sales, from our hotel in Hawaii to the Sandalwood Farm. It's about a 90-minute ride. Young Living had pre-arranged for one of the execs to ride on each of the four or five buses our group took that day. They each shared stories from the trenches, talked about the oils, passed out prizes (a graciously generous amount!), and passed the time with us. It was an incredible experience- and, yes, Gary Young, himself rode on a bus!

I found out during the ride (there and back, a total of three hours) that Scott is a walking "essential oil encyclopedia." He looks like a normal guy. Goes by "Scott" instead of "Doctor." He uses everyday language instead of words with more than five syllables. Looks more like a triathlete, than a professor with his shaved head and a lean body. But he clearly knows his stuff.

So when he said, "Everything that's labelled *'essential oil'* is not necessarily the same," from the stage the morning of Nature's Remedies, I perked up. I expected Scott to launch into a scientific explanation to further explain. However, Scott explained that some companies aren't even trying to deceive you when they label their products as "pure." Some clearly are, but others "honestly have a different idea of what a pure oil is and what an adulterated oil is," Scott continued.

Then he showed us an example straight from some correspondence.[135] A French exporter had contacted Young Living about selling his oils. Because Young Living is the world industry leader in essential oils, this type of thing happens quite regularly.

"The distiller proposed to sell Young Living a 100% pure lavender oil," Scott explained. "Then the gentleman defined what *pure* meant to him."

The man's definition read as follows: "(50% lavender & 50% lavandin) 100% pure."

You don't have to know trig or calculus to understand that 50% of one thing and 50% of another is not 100% of one thing. It's *not* pure. It's cut. By half.

Again, the man sending the proposal wasn't trying to deceive anyone- he was being honest about what he was offering to sell. At the end of the day, though,

---

[135] "Core Vigor and Vitality" (in *School of Nature's Remedies* series), p5. The email text is included on that page.

his definition of pure is different than yours and mine. And **that makes a huge difference when you're talking about what an essential oil can do- what those tiny traveling super-concentrated power-houses that can raise your frequency levels are capable of**.

Scott also explained to us that lavandin, the added ingredient the salesman was using, sometimes causes skin irritation. Lavandin is a cross between lavender and spike lavender- and it contains a compound known as camphor.[136] Lavender is often used to stop bleeding and to heal cuts, scrapes, and even burns. If you put lavandin on a cut, though, the camphor might cause inflammation.[137] This would lead you to think that essential oils simply "don't work," when the issue wasn't the lavender at all- it was the extra ingredient.

> ... your natural state is health and wholeness. Your body, when healthy is fighting for health- not fighting for disease. Your body, when healthy and whole, is moving higher in frequency.

Scott mentioned another scenario that plays out when potential suppliers call Young Living.[138] Young Living will often say something like, "Sure, send us a sample. We'll test it in our lab and get back to you."

The next question that often comes from the vendor is, "What do you want it to *smell* like?"

Scott offered the hypothetical response that YL kicks back, *"What do you mean, 'What do we want it to smell like?' We want it to smell like what it smells like!"*

I've smelled over 120 of the oils. My wife earned an aroma complete kit worth $1,900 chock full of oils for hitting the "Silver in Six" mark as a distributor. The day the oils arrived, we sat in the living room and smelled *all* of them. Honestly, I love how some of them smell. Others... well... let's just say I didn't care for.

But the *Young Living oils all smell like what they should smell like.* That's an odd sentence, I know, but I'm trying to communicate to you that the oils smell like whatever the plant produces. They don't smell like a preferred scent that

---

[136] The man was selling a blend- and not a single oil. He was not selling a synthetic.

[137] Source: Scott Johnson, private message, 04-07-2014.

[138] Scott Johnson, opening session, Nature's Remedies conference, March 22, 2014. BJCC.

someone created in a lab and then injected into the oils, thereby diluting it, and making it more pleasant to the olfactory palette.

This leads me to a major point about oils: **all essential oils are *not* created equally**. The *Essential Oils Pocket Reference* contrasts two qualities of essential oils: *aromatherapy* grade and *therapeutic* grade.

Aromatherapy grade oils are cheaper than therapeutic grade oils. They are watered-down, the essential parts of them are stretched to fill more bottles, and they have added fillers (i.e., fragrances). You can't ingest them, and the label on the bottle will say so.

Because of all of the additives, you have weakened their ability to travel, you have bonded things to them and made them larger than they should be, you have lowered their frequency, and you have paid good money to do it. Not as much as you pay for legit, full strength oils, but still…

Therapeutic grade oils, on the other hand, are *pure*. There is nothing added to them at all. You only get the aromatic, volatile substance of the original plant. Therefore, you can actually ingest many therapeutic grade oils (i.e., you can place drops of it in a capsule and swallow it, you can drop it in water/rice milk and drink it). You should *never* do that with a lower-grade oil, however. (And as a side note: Not all therapeutic grade oils *should* be ingested. Young Living always recommends consulting with your primary medical care provider before ingesting therapeutic grade essential oils if you are pregnant, nursing or have other medical conditions.)

You need to research the oil producer and find out if, like the Frenchman in the lavender example above, his definition of pure is the same as yours. Some manufacturers promote their oils as "pure" when they clearly aren't. Again, sometimes this is intentional deception, sometimes it's not. I'm not getting into their motivations for doing this, I'm simply stating the raw fact.

To be clear, "Young Living offers pure and authentic oils *as close to how they are found in their natural and living state as possible.*"[139] By contrast, Daniel Penoel, who writes the forward for Gary's book *An Introduction to Young Living Essential Oils*, says, "Many companies have jumped onto the *aromatic bandwagon* solely for commercial reasons. They simply do not know the meaning of genuine when it is applied to essential oils. They market products that are made solely for what I call *recreational fragrancing.*"[140]

---

[139] "Core Vigor and Vitality" (in *School of Nature's Remedies* series), p5.

[140] Gary Young, *An Introduction to Young Living Essential Oils*, iii.

Recreational fragrancing? Yes, recreational. As such, I would add a third category of oils: *novelty* grade.

There's a shop in 5 Points South near downtown Birmingham, a local intersection that has a few clubs, a coffee shop, several restaurants, and an undefined shop where you can purchase old records, hipster clothes, and drug paraphernalia- for "display purposes only," of course.

They sell incense sticks in that shop at the meager price of "5 for $1.00." Light them, and the smells rises with a tiny, winding smoke stream. You can buy cinnamon sticks, peppermint, lemongrass, patchouli, juniper, and fennel- among other types. Yep, the same names as the essential oils that Young Living manufactures.

> Because of all of the additives, you have weakened their ability to travel, you have bonded things to them and made them larger than they should be, you have lowered their frequency, and you have paid good money to do it.

There is nothing "essential" about any of those sticks. They smell good, but they don't qualify as aromatherapeutic or therapeutic. They're *novelty*. Period. It doesn't make them bad- it just means that not everything that has the name of an essential oil is worthy of the name "essential oil."

Why would someone alter the oils? Here are a few obvious reasons:

- Your profit margin is higher if you can stretch the product.

- More people will buy a cheaper product (who wants to spend $10.00 on a single incense stick when they can buy *five* for $1.00?).

- Your shelf life is longer (food people have known this for years- hence, all the additives and preservatives).

- You can control the final product.

Remember, a few pages ago I mentioned to you that the essential oils contain the "life force" of the original plant. I know, it sounds New Age or Star Wars-ish, but once you understand the truth of it, a lot of things start making complete sense. You start understanding why the oils work.[141] And you start really seeing why you want pure oils instead of half-breeds. Or even non-breeds.

Yes, there are oils on the market that are 100% synthetic. That's *not* an essential oil, even though it may be marketed as such. As you become more and more familiar with oils and how they are derived, you'll see that "a large percentage of essential oils marketed in the United States fall in this adulterated category."[142]

This leads me back to Gary and the calloused hands that I shook the first time I met him in Hawaii. Find a guy who is serious about quality- so much so that 34 percent of the oil samples submitted to him from May 2007 to October 2011 were rejected- and you start seeing the difference in a major way.[143] Use the oils, and the difference becomes even clearer.

The Seed to Seal process

Young Living has a special process that is so unique to them that they've actually trademarked it. It's call the "Seed to Seal" guarantee and means that there is a documented chain of custody from the time the seed is acquired to the time it goes into the ground, is grown, matures, is harvested, then distilled, and finally makes it into a bottle wrapped with their label. They certify that each bottle that with the Young Living seal has passed throughout their strict requirements for purity and quality and they can account for it at some specific farm that they either own or maintain a partnering relationship.[144]

Here's what the process looks like:

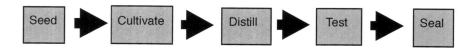

---

[141] Here's an example from the Bible. Re-read the passages about animal sacrifice, and notice how often frankincense is involved. When you understand that frankincense eradicates disease from blood and brings cleansing, you get a glimpse into why God instructed it to be part of the offerings. The frankincense would protect the people- and the priests- from catching any disease. This is also why frankincense is so effective in treating cancer.

[142] *Essential Oils Desk Reference*, Fifth Edition, location 1.4.

[143] *Essential Oils Pocket Reference*, p18.

[144] www.YoungLiving.com/en_US/discover/quality

Let's walk through it.

Step #1- Seed

If you build your house on the wrong foundation, it won't stand- no matter how much care you take with framing the house and the paint job on the final product. The same is true in the Seed to Seal process. You must start with the right thing in the beginning or your later efforts are in vain.

The seeds must come from the right genus, as well as the correct species. If the seed is bad, it doesn't matter how much correct cultivation you do- or what the packaging looks like when the bottle is displayed in your medicine cabinet.

> "Young Living offers pure and authentic oils *as close to how they are found in their natural and living state as possible.*"

For Young Living's purposes, this means that clove oil may come from Madagascar, citrus arrives from Spain, Helichrysum imports from Corsica, and Sandalwood will now also come from Hawaii.[145] Furthermore, Gary is constantly studying new plants in new locations.

Recently, this led him undercover to Somalia, where he was snuck in- and raced out. Yes, his life was in danger- and his wife probably had a conversation with him that we'd all love to hear. But that's how he is- he's a mover and a shaker.

Because you can't really manufacture the true essence of an oil by creating a plant in a greenhouse or other controlled environment. Young Living goes to where the plant is and obtains that plant on the plants own terms. Young Living hand plants acres and acres of seeds. They nourish the soils with "enzymes, minerals, and organic mulch," realizing that the "content of the soil is crucial to the proper development of the plant."[146] Indeed, "soils that lack minerals result in plants that produce inferior oils."[147]

---

[145] *Essential Oils Desk Reference*, location 1.38.

[146] *Essential Oils Desk Reference*, location 1.39.

[147] *Essential Oils Desk Reference*, location 1.39.

Step #2- Cultivate

After the seed has established itself in the ground, what you do with it remains of equal importance. Cultivation is vital. Think of it like raising a kid; you may have an incredible birth experience, but if you don't take care of the child for the next 18 years or so something's going to go amiss! I know, plants aren't as important as people, but you get the idea here.

As I just mentioned, the country of origin is often important. In some locations (i.e., Idaho), the plants are cultivated and grown by Young Living's personnel. In other countries around the world, the plants are grown through partnerships that Young Living has established. The majority of these partners have decades of experience with specific plants. They know what proper growing conditions are needed, the optimal times for harvesting (some plants are best harvested in the middle of the night!). In many cases, their families have been "in the business" for generations.

A lot of experience and forethought go into proper cultivation. Young Living has purposed that their plants "should be grown on virgin land uncontaminated by chemical fertilizers, pesticides, fungicides, or herbicides. They should also be grown away from nuclear plants, factories, interstates, highways, and heavily-populated cities, if possible."[148]

> Think of it like raising a kid; you may have an incredible birth experience, but if you don't take care of the child for the next 18 years or so something's going to go amiss!

They've decided that plants should be watered from wells, reservoirs, mountain streams, and water-sheds instead of municipally treated water that contains numerous chemicals and toxins. Naturally-occurring water sources are cleaner, purer, and usually have a high mineral content.

Young Living maintains standards for cultivation that are higher than any other criteria you will find. The USDA does certify items as "natural" and "organic." Certain criteria must be met in order for producers to label their foods "certified organic" at the supermarket. However, these labels (though they are great to look for) focus only on growing in a natural environment that is *free of chemicals and toxins.* Such labels do not account for the time of harvest, quality of the soil or extraction methods used. As well, they do not account for the environment in which something was originally *seeded* and *cultivated* (the first two of the five

---

[148] *Essential Oils Desk Reference*, location 1.39.

categories in the Seed to Seal process). Because there is ongoing debate surrounding the use of GMO products in the cultivation process, it's likely the seal of "organic" is even more unreliable than originally thought.[149]

A truly natural approach, such as Young Living's Seed to Seal, takes into consideration that cultivation is absolutely vital to the health of their plants and thus their oils. All essential oils are somewhat different, even from the same plant from the same genus and species of seed. Because climates change, soil conditions are different, and the harvest from year to year will look somewhat unique to the previous year's- even in the exact same location you will find a slightly varied end result with each harvest. "Plants inherently have varying degrees of compounds in them based on harvest time, growing type, geographic region, etc."[150]

Step #3- Distill

Cultivation reaches completion and the plant is harvested. Then, comes the distillation process. And then we finally get to see what we've been waiting for: the oil.

Distilling is very much a science and an art form. Because of the great deal of specificity surrounding the entire process, distillation is quite complex. Gary expounds that "Essential oils can be extracted from different parts of the plants or trees, such as seeds, flowers, petals, stems, roots, bark, or even the whole plant. It is even possible for different oils to be extracted from one single tree or plant."[151]

He goes on to describe how, with the orange tree, the peel is processed for orange oil, the leaves and twigs are used for petitgraine oil, and the blossoms are used for neroli oil. All three oils are incredibly useful for therapeutic purposes.[152] Only a trained cultivator and distiller would know this, though. Someone else might waste useful parts of the tree- or simply toss everything

---

[149] *Essential Oils Desk Reference*, Fifth Edition, location 1.37.

[150] Scott Johnson, *Surviving When Modern Medicine Fails*, p9.

[151] *Aromatherapy*, Gary Young, p20.

[152] *Aromatherapy*, Gary Young, p20.

into one distiller and make a single oil that would be less potent for a specific purpose.

As well, distillers must use the ideal cuttings of the part of the plant they are distilling. For example, the bud of the clove plant is the part used for distilling. If you put the entire plant in, your essential oil will not contain the proper chemical constituents.

Oddly enough, even *the time of day* in which plants are harvested can be one of the most important factors that determines the grade of oil that is produced. The *Essential Oils Desk Reference* reads, "If the plants are harvested at the wrong time of the season or even at the incorrect time of day, they may distill into a substandard essential oil."[153] And, "… if the plants are distilled… with incorrect distillation procedures, the compounds that make the oils therapeutic will not be there."[154]

The reference book provides a specific example, noting that "changing harvest time, *by even a few hours*, can make a huge difference. For example, German chamomile harvested in the morning will produce oil with far more azulene (a powerful anti-inflammatory compound) than chamomile harvested in late afternoon."[155]

The amount of dew that is present, the percentage of plant that is in bloom, and even the weather the few weeks leading to harvest time all effect the oil that is produced. As well, distillers must know how many times to distill the plant. I read that "essential oils can be distilled or extracted in different ways that will have dramatic effects on their chemistry and medicinal action. Oils derived from a second or third distillation of the same plant material are usually not as potent as oils extracted during the first distillation."[156] This might lead you to believe that the "first run" is always the best. However, "with certain oils, there may be additional chemical constituents that are released only in the second or third distillation."[157]

In addition to harvesting standards, Young Living purposes to have distillation facilities as close to the fields as possible. They believe that transporting

---

[153] *Essential Oils Desk Reference*, location 1.39.

[154] *Essential Oils Pocket Reference*, p18.

[155] *Essential Oils Desk Reference*, location 1.39, emphasis added.

[156] *Essential Oils Desk Reference*, Fifth Edition, location 1.4.

[157] *Essential Oils Desk Reference*, Fifth Edition, location 1.4.

harvested plant material to facilities days of travel time away elevates the risk of pollution, contamination, and mold.[158] And because essential oils are the life force of the plant, the fresher the plant the more it produces a more vibrant and life-giving oil.

While we where in Hawaii, the farmers there told us the optimal time to harvest Royal Hawaiian Sandalwood was *after it died*. Notably, this is a different time than when other Sandalwoods throughout the world are distilled,

> ...because essential oils are the life force of the plant, the fresher the plant the more it produces a more vibrant and life-giving oil.

again echoing the fact that every plant and every climate is incredibly unique. In keeping with Young Living's standard, the distilling equipment for the Sandalwood was on-site. We literally walked a few hundred yards from the place where we planted new trees to the spot where distillation occurs.

Step #4- Test

While Young Living is committed to ensuring a top-notch plant that will produce a high-grade oil, they don't just *assume* the process worked according to plan. They go the extra mile and test each lot sample using their state-of-the-art equipment, checking them against time-tested markers for that specific oil. This testing equipment costs hundreds of thousands of dollars. However, Young Living does not stop there. The company also sends the oils to third party laboratories for *more* testing and verification.

Right now, "The European communities have tight controls and standards concerning botanical extracts and who may administer them."[159] That is, you can't just call something a "pure oil" and start peddling it. In Europe, anyway. Currently, the United States does *not* have a regulatory agency that oversees the creation, distribution, and use of essential oils- such as the FDA that oversees food and drugs.[160] In the U.S., then, anyone can set up shop, sell essential oils and call themselves an aromatherapist. You don't need any training- you don't

---

[158] For a lengthy explanation of distillation, see the *Essential Oils Desk Reference*, chapter 5, "Producing Therapeutic-Grade Essential Oils."

[159] *Essential Oils Desk Reference*, Fifth Edition, location 1.3.

[160] I'm not arguing for or against the FDA- I'm just stating that no such thing exists for oils!

even have to have read the book.[161] You just need a sign and a few oils. Furthermore, you don't even have to provide *good* quality oils. You can use anything you desire.

Young Living has raised the bar in the U.S. as to what qualifies as a therapeutic grade essential oil. Gary and his crew were "the first to establish guidelines that define what a therapeutic essential oil is and to create oils that met or exceeded any known medicinal standard."[162] This all happens via the Seed to Seal process.

Step #5- Seal

Here's an important point: the oil is sealed and then shipped, and it is labelled as it is for what it is. I know, that's an odd sentence. Here's what it means: there's integrity in the process.

"Literally, from the plant seed that is dropped into the soil to the essential oil sealed in the amber bottle in Young Living's state-of-the-art bottling facility, the Seed-to-Seal process is carefully supervised from beginning to end to ensure quality and purity of Young Living Therapeutic-Grade essential oils."[163]

Lately, there's been some contention surrounding oils that are "shipped from Oman." Particularly, Frankincense. Young Living oils all follow the Seed to Seal process- so the oil you get from Oman is from plants that have been seeded, cultivated, distilled, tested, and then sealed in Oman. That's why the bottles denote that they are from Oman.

I don't know of any other manufacturer of essential oils that has a process rivaling Young Living's unique Seed to Seal approach. This means that something labeled as shipped from Oman may mean just that- it was *shipped* from Oman. Not "grown in Oman."

When Cristy and I flew back from the Drive to Win Hawaii trip, we chose to have a lay-over in Portland instead of flying the red-eye. We figured with nine kids waiting for us back in Birmingham, we'd better have our "A-game" on when we

---

[161] For more detail on this dilemma see *Essential Oils Desk Reference*, Fifth Edition, location 1.4.

[162] *Essential Oils Desk Reference*, Fifth Edition, location 1.37.

[163] See page7 of "Core Vigor and Vitality," in *School of Nature's Remedies*.

arrived home. Oddly enough, we ran into our friends Steven and Shellina at the Atlanta airport. They'd just come back from somewhere in Europe.

"We flew in from Portland," we said. Technically, it was true and not true. We flew in from Hawaii via Portland. We didn't do anything in Portland at all. It was a mere stop on the way.

Some essential oils are like that. They ship "from" various parts of the world in the same way that we came in from Washington. We didn't *really* come from Portland- we just stayed there the night.

> They cost a bit more than other lesser oils, but they pack a lot more powerful punch.

Here's your question if you think you have an oil that simply "spent the night" as opposed to actually "came from" somewhere: Where was it planted? Where was it distilled? Who tested it? How was it sealed? Was it even sealed at all? What is the *chain of custody* for the product?

Now you know why Young Living oils *seem* relatively expensive. Quite simply, "producing pure oils is very costly."[164] I mentioned earlier in the chapter that it required a great amount of plant matter to produce a relatively small amount of oil- if the oil is pure. They cost a bit more than other lesser oils, but they pack a lot more powerful punch.

By the way, here's a few numbers that will make you look smart. Young Living offers 90 different oils and 71 different blends that run through this Seed to Seal process.[165] That's 161 current oils all working through that Seed to Seal process.

Back full circle

A perfect illustration of Young Living's Seed to Seal guarantee can be found by looking at Haloa Aina, Young Living's newest partner farm. This breathtaking farm rests at one of the highest elevations on the Big Island of Hawaii.

Jeff Lee is one of the owners and serves as the managing partner, where he's merged his skill of management with his love of Hawaii and her people. He and his wife own a successful health club near Kona, where they teach exercise as

[164] *Essential Oils Desk Reference*, Fifth Edition, location 1.46.

[165] "Core Vigor and Vitality" (in *School of Nature's Remedies* series), p7.

part of an overall lifestyle of health and wholeness. Jeff is tan and athletic, and looks like he could lead a cross fit class, run any piece of heavy machinery on a farm, or teach a college class. He's a man a many talents.

We gathered at his farm during our trip to Hawaii to learn about Royal Hawaiian Sandalwood- one of the next oils to be released by Young Living. Jeff was standing at the end of a large, white canopy tent that had been erected to provide meeting space in the open air for the 100 or so of us that gathered.

"By the way," Jeff told the group, "Hawaii is said to be named after the Polynesian explorer who first came here…"

Jeff explained to us that Hawaii was home to various chiefs and fiefdoms in the late 1700s- back in the age of discovery.

…after decades of Westernization and other sociological shifts the pieces of pie are no longer whole, but the idea of working together and sustaining the land remains.

"A warrior named Kamehameha was able to finally unify the island in 1810," Jeff continued.

Apparently, this unifying king divided the Big Island like a pie- and the different clans and groups that had once fought each other were each given a slice. Like a pie, each slice started at the center of the island, and worked out to the coast.

"Each family group had a piece of coast… and a piece of the mountains," he taught us, "and we learned that we all had to live together and care for one another. No more fighting. No more bickering. Just working and living together."

Haloa Aina sits in the tract that has been in Jeff's family for centuries, and crowns the top of their historic piece of pie. Yes, after decades of Westernization and other sociological shifts the pieces of pie are no longer whole, but the idea of working together and sustaining the land remains.

"This farm is 2,800 acres. It stretches…" Jeff said, painting broad landmarks with his arms in the air, tracing the property lines "… up to the top of this hill…" He pointed to the hill where the distillation equipment sits in an open-air metal canopy that looks likes an over-sized carport. "… to the bottom of the hills here…" and he pointed towards where the coast might be…

That's six square miles of wild forest recovery. Six square miles of land that is being reclaimed. Six square miles of *peace* and *bliss* and *calm*. At some point within the first 15 minutes of being there and listening to Jeff, we all learned that our cell phones didn't work anymore. We'd lost the coverage about 2 miles back down the hill. It was a nice change. No phone. No email. Just nature and lots of people who love each other and what they do.

The reforestation project is home to the *Santalum Paniculatum* tree. You know it as Royal Hawaiian Sandalwood. Jeff, his family, and a small crew of others have been laboring the land since 2009. At that time, the land was almost barren.

"The Sandalwood had been traded throughout the entire world, dating back to the 1790s," Jeff taught us, "back in the days of exploration, when the first Polynesians came to the Big Island."

Then he cracked a joke- a joke that rang of great truth. "The Main Landers came over and brought their ways with them... that about ended the Sandalwood trade..."

Apparently, the Main Landers (the name they use for those from the *Main Land*- the continental United States- decided the hill we were standing on would be great for cattle. So the cattle came, they burrowed into the trees, and they stripped them of their bark. What was once a profitable Sandalwood trade was replaced by a different profitable- and more destructive- trade as the beef industry began edging its way into the culture.

Jeff and his organization have been reforesting the area. They've had tremendous success in a relatively short time. 200,000 trees now fill the landscape, making it the most dense Sandalwood reservation in the world. When fully grown, some of them will stand 50 feet tall, and span 30 or more feet. Most will stand slightly smaller.[166]

> Gary suggested we might be- that we depend on what we find on the earth to sustain us. In turn, we must care for that earth so that it continues. Oddly enough, our sustainability is in sustaining it.

Remarkably, *none of the trees will grow and stand on their own,* though. At one point while Jeff was talking, he looked to Gary- somehow giving him the nod to continue the conversation.

---

[166] http://haloaaina.com/sustainable-forestry-products-royal-hawaiian-sandalwood-oil says, "The variety used by Haloa Aina Royal Hawaiian Sandalwood, *Santalum Paniculatum*, is endemic to Hawaii Island (the Big Island) and found in a montane (4,000 to 7,000ft) dry environment Mamane and Naio forest with scattered Koa and an understory of various native shrubs including Pukiawe, Lauala, and Aali'i. Our Big Island climate is ideal and these sandalwood trees can reach over 50 feet high with a canopy diameter of over 30 feet, aver- age trees are 33 feet high and have canopies measuring around 23 feet" (accessed 03-25-2014).

"Sandalwood is a parasite," Gary said. That sounds like an odd statement, but he then elaborated on something that Jeff had described to us earlier. Jeff taught the group that Sandalwood trees grow up intertwining themselves with other trees.

"Everyone wants to grow Sandalwood," Jeff said. "People have used it for religious reasons… Ghandi is said to have been burned atop 4,000 pounds of Sandalwood, even though it's very expensive." Then he hit the nail on the head- "The problem," he mentioned, "is that people *only* want Sandalwood…"

But you can't have Sandalwood *alone*. "To get Sandalwood you must plant and grow the entire forest. That way you get Sandalwood- but it comes with everything else!"

This is what Gary was talking about. "Sandalwood grows with the rest of the forest," Gary said. And- "It's dependent on other things and *leans* on other things for its survival…"

Aren't we parasites, too? Gary suggested we might be- that we depend on what we find on the earth to sustain us. In turn, we must care for that earth so that it continues. Oddly enough, our sustainability is in sustaining it.

In all of this **I found myself thinking more and more like an environmentalist but from a standpoint that sees *the purpose* behind it all**- not just saving the earth because it's our "mother" or because it's the latest bumper sticker slogan to put on a t-shirt or coffee mug or FaceBook post, but because some of the first words God said to us were to steward the earth, that it had been given to us to use, but that it had to be managed- not just stripped.

We walked from about 400 yards to the top of the mountain, to the place where the Sandalwood is distilled.

"Wind comes down at night, whipping through the open front and back of the large metal canopy. The workers set some of the logs aside to sell. It will become trim in high-end homes and furniture that sits in offices. The wood that is too small for those uses will become mulch," Jeff described.

He lifted some of the mulch in his hand whilst standing atop a pile of it. Our group stood gathered around him, three or four deep in a large semi-circle. Some stooped to grab a handful of the mulch, others sat atop the distiller.

"The best oil comes from the roots," he said. "And it comes from the most distressed trees." Then, "It's almost like the tree secretes the oil when it's under duress... like that's when the most beautiful part- and the most healing part- of the plant is created... when trouble comes."

He paused. He laughed. "That's just like life, isn't it? You look back and can tell when these trees went through a tough season... a famine... or a sickness... or something else... because of when the healing power came and the beautiful oils were created. We're much the same, aren't we...?"

During this meeting beside the distillery, Gary shared that his involvement with Sandalwood goes back a few years. He told us that he originally had a crew cut down an old, dying tree in another country.

"Now lay it down on the side," he said- so they did.

Then he instructed them to cut the root ball off and load it on a shipping container at the dock. They thought he was crazy when he asked for the tree. They *knew* he was crazy when he asked for the roots of that ragged tree.

Gary took the root ball to Idaho, to the distillation plant, and he began to work his magic. Then he took the final product to Mary, who he lovingly referred to as his guinea pig. He swears she is better than any R & D department, and that she is far more skilled at spotting a superior oil than any of the fancy machines.

After applying it to her face, "It's the best Sandalwood I've ever tried!" she exclaimed.

With the wife's nod of approval, Gary began running the tests, knowing what they would confirm. The best essential oil of sandalwood is found in the root system and the older the tree, the better.

> Some of the first words God said to us were to steward the earth, that it had been given to us to use, but that it had to be managed- not just stripped.

And then came the *big unveil*. A beautiful bottle of Young Living branded and labeled Royal Hawaiian Sandalwood. "Many people prefer Royal Hawaiian Sandalwood to other varieties of Sandalwood we produce from Sri Lanka," Gary told us, as he introduced the new oil to us in Hawaii.

In Sri Lanka and in India, Sandalwood grows at 500 feet above sea level. We were standing at 5,000 feet above the oceans that you could see in the distance there on the Big Island- 10 times the optimal elevation for other types of Sandalwood. Somehow, the altitude actually helps the efficacy of the soil in Hawaii's oil.

Hawaiian Sandalwood is also unique because of the lava tubes that fill the island's terrain. I had noticed the previous day when Cristy and I were walking along the beach that the oceanfront wasn't at all like the sandy dunes we have on the Gulf. Rather, the coast of the Big Island is covered with charcoal-black chunks of dried and cooled lava.

Several active volcanoes remain in the area, and it is not uncommon to see miles of road where people had gathered the bright white coral from the ocean and placed in on the dark lava to spell out their name in giant four and five foot tall letters. Jack loves Jill. Congratulations, Phil. Happy Anniversary... such messages dot the roads that connect town to town along the coastal areas.

The lava tubes at the top of the mountains are important to the Sandalwood tree's survival. "They create a sort of eco system in which the trees thrive," Jeff told us. "The Sandalwood grows down into lava tubes, the roots stretch through the tunnels, and they absorb the gases and the minerals from the lava."

Before the day wrapped, our group spread across the rugged Hawaiian terrain in three large groups. Some of us planted young saplings. Others erected protection boundaries around young trees that were beginning to form. Others gathered seeds.

We left with a bottle of Young Living's Royal Hawaiian Sandalwood- something that wouldn't be available for purchase for several more months.

> The leaves of the trees *are* for the healing of the nations.

Cristy and I had the privilege of spending some one on one time with Jeff and his lovely wife Marlena later that evening at Gary's suite as they meandered throughout our group. I remember him telling us, "They're harvesting Sandalwood as quick as 12 years in Australia," he said. Then- "But the trees here in Hawaii can grow for 70 years..." He detailed how the Sandalwood trees in various continents and climates are of a different species.

"70 years!" I replied. "Amazing." Then I added, "You're building something that you won't ever see."

He grinned. "I know," he said with his large smile. "That's why nobody else is doing it."

And there it is full circle. We've been given stewardship over the land. The land has what we need for health and healing. For wholeness. For life. So we should use it.

But if we don't replenish it, there won't be any left for others to use.[167] Even for the people we may never meet.

Young Living's commitment to the environment and sustainability is unmatched by any other company. They believe that producing a therapeutic grade oil begins with a heart for the land, her plant and soil and for the people who steward it. The leaves of the trees *are* for the healing of the nations.

---

[167] Yes, this means letting the Sandalwood grow its life cycle- and then die- without cutting it prematurely. It also means planting more Sandalwood. It's not an "either / or" proposition, but a "both / and."

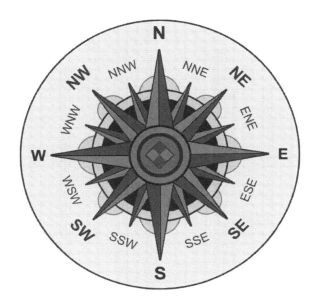

03: Direction: learn a little

Action steps

Main idea: Essentials oils are a small, unique part of each plant. They are, in a sense, part of the life force of that plant, each plant having a unique version of its own.

☐ Get the names of 5 of the oils- ones that you will actually use for yourself. Write down what they do, and how you can use them.

   ☐ Oil #1

      ☐ What: _____

      ☐ How to use it: _____

   ☐ Oil #2

      ☐ What: _____

      ☐ How to use it: _____

☐ Oil #3

    ☐ What: _____

    ☐ How to use it: _____

☐ Oil #4

    ☐ What: _____

    ☐ How to use it: _____

☐ Oil #5

    ☐ What: _____

    ☐ How to use it: _____

☐ Why does Proverbs 21:20 say that "the house of the wise has stores of oil" inside?[168]

Want to know more?

☐ Read:

    ☐ "How Do Essential Oils Work?" Chapter 4 in *Aromatherapy: The Essential Beginning*, by D. Gary Young

    ☐ "How Essential Oils Work," Chapter 2 in *An Introduction to Young Living Essential Oils*, by D. Gary Young

    ☐ "Frequency of Essential Oils," Chapter 5 in *Aromatherapy: The Essential Beginning*, by D. Gary Young

    ☐ "Frequency and Distillation," Chapter 3 *An Introduction to Young Living Essential Oils*, by D. Gary Young

---

[168] David Stewart raises this question in *Healing Oils of the Bible*, p280.

☐ "How Essential Oils Work," Chapter 2 in *Essential Oils Pocket Reference*, Life Science Publishing[169]

☐ "How and Why Oils Can Heal," Chapter 2 in *Healing Oils of the Bible*, David Stewart

☐ *Surviving When Modern Medicine Fails,* Scott Johnson. This entire book is one long, flowing chapter. Pages 5-14 deal with essential oils and their backgrounds. This is helpful reading. Treatment protocols follow, beginning at page 15.

☐ "Core Vigor and Vitality" (in *School of Nature's Remedies* series)

☐ Listen:

☐ To the relevant chapter of the audiobook

☐ Search:

☐ Review the "Seed to Seal" process at Young Living's website: www.YoungLiving.com/en_US/discover/quality

☐ Review the website for *Haloa Aina*, the Hawaiian Sandalwood farm: www.haloaaina.com

---

[169] I have referenced this book a few times. It is a condensed version of a larger book, *Essential Oils Desk Reference* (also compiled by Life Science Publishing). If you want to study more about natural health, go to the desk reference. It adds additional information about supplements and health.

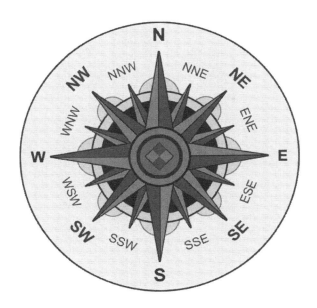

03: Out of my comfort zone / Stephen's story

As a natural skeptic, I was not supportive of my wife's first description of essential oils. When I think of the idea of "holistic medicine," the first things that comes to mind are hippies, wives' tales, new age

Stephen Hall has been married to Kelly for almost 17 years. They have three biological kids and welcome foster children into their home. Kelly has been a distributor for Young Living since September 2013.

freaks, and Scientologists. If you told me a year ago, that I would use essential oils for health purposes, I would have called you crazy... or worse. However, through the last five months, I have come to realize their benefits and effectiveness.

My story is pretty simple. We tried essential oils, found great success, and became avid users. Success happened immediately. My 10 year old son is a soccer player who was struggling with knee pain. Our doctor advised us to give him Ibuprofen on a regular schedule. Since that drug can potentially cause harm to the liver, we became a little concerned. Adding Ibuprofen to his regular schedule of acid reflux and allergy medicines put me in a place where I was giving my son quite a bit of medicine each day.

Being hopeful, we rubbed Panaway oil on our son's knee. It worked better than Ibuprofen. Since that time, we have gotten him off allergy medicine and acid reflux medicine, as well. These are only some of the impressive results we have had with our family.

I must admit we affectionately refer to my wife as a witchdoctor. My brother-in-law jokingly refers to the oils as "snake oils," but knows the results speak for themselves. The kids and I have enjoyed harassing her and her "voodoo" practices.

However, the fruit is the proof.

It seems that people are daily asking her for oil advice and coming by our house for samples. She loves helping others. Of course watching her make capsules of oils for friends lead us to continue to see her as the neighborhood "witch doctor."

Honestly, I am surprised that I have found success in using oils. For a while, I tried to convince myself that oils produce nothing more than a placebo affect.

As a conservative theologian and a Southern Baptist minister, I would have thought that I would be least likely to be in complete agreement with the use of essential oils. However, I have had success curbing my own acid reflux, as well (it runs in the family- or, at least, it used to).

We have drastically decreased the amount of medicine our family consumes. My wife has spent hours of time researching and learning about essential oils, regularly hosting classes and teaching others.

For quite a while, I looked on skeptically. However, I have seen legitimate results and I have learned about the solid research and science behind the use of oils. The time for suspicion is over. This stuff is legit.

— Stephen Hall, Kelly's husband

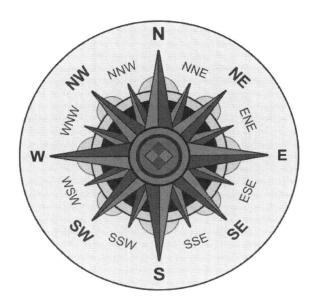

04: How I got here

I told you earlier that Cristy and I never intended to make money as distributors with Young Living. She simply wanted to make enough money to "pay for her own."

We've been using herbal remedies and essential oils for years, for over a decade. We were told about Young Living about 8 years ago and were actually talked out of buying them- *by a distributor*- due to the cost of YL as opposed to lesser grade oils.

The main idea: If you have a kit- or, more accurately if your wife does- you're already a distributor. Whether you do anything with it is up to you. Get comfortable with the possibilities…

Cristy is a childbirth educator, and she is a doula liaison for the natural birth community at one of the largest hospitals in the State of Alabama. We birthed four of our biological kids with a Certified Professional Midwife in the home birth setting- three of them as water births. Things that are *natural* are not new to us.

Even so, I didn't know much of anything about essential oils until the past few months. I gave you a lot of information about what they are and how they work in the previous chapter. I'm *just now* learning all of that.

I know that we've used Arnica, a homeopathic remedy, to alleviate bruises and swelling. I know that we've used Eucalyptus oil to ease chest congestion and coughs, and we've used herbal elderberry to fight viruses. I've used a vaporizer before- but never a *diffuser*. We've done those things for years. But until the past month I've not been overly health conscious. I relayed to you earlier that Cristy pretty much handled "all things Young Living" in our household by herself without much input or interest from me for the first six months.

For the past few years, I've pretty much eaten whatever I wanted to, gone back for seconds, and then managed my weight (read: *gained weight at a slower rate than I would have*) by exercising about three or four times a week. My kids knew to ask me if they wanted pizza or some form of junk food, instead of asking their mom. Especially donuts. Particularly "baby angels."[170]

One day the girls saw a stack of soda cans in our pantry floor. "Thanks, Dad!" they exclaimed.

"For what?"

"For the Cokes," they said. Just so you know… in the South we label any soda a *coke*. It's become a generic term- not just a brand.

"I didn't get them for you," I replied. Then, "I guess Mom did!"

"That's *really weird*," Ivey, our second oldest, replied.

She was in *shock*. Disbelief. Bringing sugary cereals and unhealthy snacks and bottles of soda into the house was something I did- not something Cristy did. That's been true for as long as I can remember- and for as long as those girls can remember, too. In fact, one of my first memories of walking my little girls through Target is when Cristy and I approached a check-out counter. Target cleverly displays 20 ounce bottled drinks at the end of their aisles, ripe for the picking.

Cristy grabbed a water- then Emma, then about 3, grabbed a Mountain Dew. "That's Daddy's juice," she said, in a matter-of-fact tone.

And it was. I would jog 4-5 miles and come in and chug a 32 ounce cup of soda. I drank it at every meal- *and more*. That changed when the Young Living lifestyle of *therapeuo* came into play.

---

[170] My kids heard comedian Tim Hawkins say that "Eating a Krispy Kreme is like eating a baby angel" and it stuck!

Enrolling as a distributor and then networking with others in the area to buy goods online and, hopefully, make enough profit to cover the cost of our own- was a normal next step for Cristy. She's been part of "co-ops" before- groups of people buying items such as organic produce, healthcare items, natural cleaning products, etc. in bulk at a cheaper price. She even handled the orders and shipping and receiving for a large group of items that used to come to our house once a month.

She also operates under the premise of "buy local" when she can. By that, I mean that she buys *even more locally* than you buy when you go to the shop down the street that sells goods that come from somewhere in our region. She'll actually buy *directly* from someone out of their house. I asked her to explain that for me, so I could relay it to you.

> Cristy *knew* that a handful of those friends would purchase with her on a monthly basis. What she didn't know is that some of them would become distributors and that her business would begin steadily growing.

"If I need make-up, I'll buy from my friend, because she's a distributor for NYR that sells make-up…" she said. "Or, if I want books for the kids, I get them from my other friend… she is a distributor for Usborne." She continued, "When I need things that my friends are selling, it just makes sense to me to buy from them, to keep my dollars local and bless others who need the income, just like we do."

We've done the same thing with jewelry and other items. We support them; they support us. In a real sense, the moms band together to help one another. We figure, *Why buy from a store with a nameless face when you can purchase directly from someone you know and love and help them provide for their family- particularly if you were going to purchase those items anyway?* She carried this same mentality into Young Living. She really thought she would tell others about the oils, then they would buy some from her if they wanted them instead of picking up aromatherapy grade oils from Whole Foods or the nearby natural market in 5 Points South.

Cristy *knew* that a handful of those friends would purchase with her on a monthly basis. What she didn't know is that some of them would become distributors and that her business would begin steadily growing. Remember, most of the people we met in Hawaii did not get into Young Living to have a business. **They got into it to simply *use* the oils like we did. In some sense, this probably made us all better distributors, though, because we came to**

love the products first rather than chasing a business opportunity. The business evolved as a natural overflow of what was happening in real life.

That doesn't mean I was onboard with the business, though. I wasn't for it or against it. I was just… well… *busy*.

The first month she started working the business side, Cristy received a check. It was for $54.03. I wasn't impressed. She was, but not me. It took a lot of work to earn $54.03. The next month, she earned a bit more- she was up to $422.34. It wasn't a life-changing sum of money, but it gave us some financial wiggle room. I started to take notice.

I asked Marty, one of the guys in our downline that you met a few chapters back when you read his story, how much money it takes to get a husband's attention. What would it take for him to see that his wife should keep spending time on this, and that he should put up with the nights away from the house, the times after 11:00 pm when he's trying to sleep but she's clicking away on the keyboard next to him in the bed…

"Less than $500 did it for me," I said. "What do you think?"

He agreed. He hadn't seen a $500 check. His wife's first check *doubled* that. "Oh, yeah. Definitely," he told me. "You can save that for a great vacation, you can buy a car. You can get new appliances since the old ones always seem to be breaking… that's a game changer."

So, Cristy had my attention at the $500 mark, but her checks continued to grow. Emma (13) and Ivey (11) both needed braces. At $3,000 per kid we were wondering how we were going to cover this.

Enter Cristy's checks.

We saved up for two commission periods and paid for Ivey's. *Cash*. No payment plan. The next month we celebrated Christmas, used some of her check for some gifts and other items we needed. The third month we paid for Emma's braces. Again *cash*.

Her business had captured my attention, so much so that (you'll laugh) I actually agreed to wear that t-shirt. Now, you see how that story fits together and where that outrageous show of support originated.

Of course, after the trip to Hawaii, after meeting Gary and feeling the culture of Young Living, after walking the farms and seeing the distillers and interacting with the incredible people who've become fast friends, I'm behind her completely. For us, Young Living is no longer a simple "side thing" that we do.

Nor is it a hobby that brings a little bit of income. It is an opportunity that we are actively seeking to grow. And here's what I'm learning: If you treat it like a hobby, you'll get paid like a hobby. If you treat it like a business, you'll get paid like a business.[171] We are beginning to see it pay like a very profitable business.

Get comfortable with multilevel marketing

Here's the deal, though, in order for Young Living to work for you, you gotta get comfortable with the fact that it's a network / multilevel / home-based marketing company. I ran into an old friend about a week ago. His wife is a distributor and we were at a Young Living event. He didn't yet know I was a distributor- or, more accurately, that I was married to one.

"Do you guys do the oils?" I asked.

He shrugged, almost apologetically. "Well… *ummm*… kind of…" He raised and lowered his hands in this see-saw motion type of thing to suggest something like "I don't know" with his non-verbals.

> If you treat it like a hobby, you'll get paid like a hobby. If you treat it like a business, you'll get paid like a business.

And remember, I know him. We've talked before. Many times. And we were at a Young Living event. And we had both *paid* to attend that event. After I explained to him that Cristy was a distributor and that she was currently doing an awesome job at both keeping our kids healthy with the oils and bringing a (significant) additional income into the house, he got comfortable talking with me. He still had questions about "Quack Watch" and some other junk he pulled from the Internet, but I was full steam into writing this book and knew enough to help encourage him in the journey.

Here's the issue that was apparent, though: *He wasn't comfortable with network marketing, so he wasn't confident with his wife's Young Living business.* Admit it. I will. You probably had your reservations about MLMs, too. I did. I had questions. Lots of them.

---

[171] Pastor James McDonald, whom I mention later in this book, first articulated this phrase in this way to me.

They'll get rich off you, but. . .

Cristy and I met Mary Young the final evening we were in Hawaii. Rumor has it that Mary is the business-mind behind everything, and that Gary's idea was simply to make the oils and get them to everyone in the best way possible. The story, which I have no idea as to whether it is true or not, is that she thought a home-based network marketing scenario would be the best delivery system. The two are an incredible team, so it makes sense that their gifts and talents might fit together this way.

Standing outside in Hawaii after a luau dinner party, Mary told us that she once found herself in the same position that you may be in. I'm not sure why she brought it up, because I was onboard by now, but I'm glad she did. Her words helped bring clarity and encouragement.

"I thought I didn't want to do it," Mary said, "that I didn't want to enroll in an MLM when I was younger. I wasn't going to join!"

She is full of energy and life. She's as enthusiastic and energetic as Gary is humbled and measured. The two of them are perfect complements to one another.

"I didn't want to do it," she repeated. "The people at the top were all going to be getting rich off of me. That's why I *refused* to do it."

It dawned on me at some point while she was talking with us that we were simply calling them "Gary and Mary." Not "Mr. Boss" and "Mrs. Boss" or any other title like that. I remembered, too, that I had to pull Travis' title out of him when speaking with him one day- and he's basically the *number two* guy on campus. There's such an unhurried and un-rushed grace with *all* of them. When they are with you, they are present to you.

Mary continued, "Sure, there's some element of truth to it. They might get rich. But you'll be getting rich, too, if they do."

Then Mary hit me with the words that solidified something in my thinking: "You've got to get comfortable with multilevel marketing."

She explained that **in a good company, the people above you can only make money if you are successful. In other words, they're motivated to help you succeed.** And, the truth is that you can *surpass* their success. You can always make more than they do. I see it happen all the time in Young Living. The person "above you" in the organization will always benefit from your success, but that success is not costing you anything.[172] And, your organization can grow faster than theirs- and you can make more money than they do. It just happens that way sometimes.

We are very grateful to Barb, Cristy's direct upline, for inviting her to attend that first informational meeting where Cristy listened to Crystal talk on that speakerphone. We hope that Cristy's success and growth blesses Barb. We want her to thrive and flourish. After all, it was Barb who invited us into this opportunity. Our lives have *dramatically* changed because of her. We've got a residual income that continues to grow. Our time is freed up. We have a vehicle in place with the possibility to help set our extended family financially (more about that later). We've travelled to Hawaii free of charge…

Think about what would happen if an employer at a regular "9 to 5" came in and said *to you*, "I'll double your salary *today*… as long as you're ok that I pay the guy who told you about this job 8% off everything you generate. It won't come out of your paycheck, I'll pay him directly"

> … in order for Young Living to work for you, you gotta get comfortable with the fact that it's a network / multilevel / home-based marketing company.

You'd be OK with that (the actual compensation for Young Living is somewhat different than a flat 8%, but it's close).[173] Somehow people get a bit squeamish when they apply the same concept to network marketing, though.

Why would I not want Barb to receive some sort of benefit? Besides, *it doesn't cost us anything* for her to get commissions on our success. Barb is a single mom, a widow, whose husband died over a decade ago. She has a great kid who is about to hit his teen years. Our success helps her as she continues to grow her own business. I hope she makes a lot of money "off us." If she makes a lot, it means we've made a lot. And she's the one who invited us to the party.

Do something that pays you more than once

I used to cut grass when I was in high school. The upside was that I made good money in a short amount of time. I could cut grass for the three months I was

---

[172] I discuss this concept in the section dealing with the compensation plan.

[173] We'll hit the compensation plan in the next chapter.

out of school for the summer and then have enough cash to fund me for the entire school year. The downside was obvious: *if I didn't work, I didn't get paid.* If at any time I quit- even for a week or so to go on vacation- the money simply stopped coming. Don't get be wrong, cutting grass is a great job. It's good because you can do it over and over and over again. The grass keeps growing, you keep cutting, and you keep collecting a paycheck.

A few friends of mine owned a store called Parkway Cleaners when I was in high school. Well, their dad did. He got into the laundry business when he got out of the army. He made a ton of money washing and ironing everyone's clothes while he was in the military. While others went on leave and took passes, he washed and folded, running his trade there in the barracks. When he got out, he used the cash to start the business that he handed off to his two boys. His hard work provided for him, for his kids, for his extended family, for their kids…

One day my dad explained to me how clever it was to start something like that cleaning business: "The guy that sells the shirt or pants get paid *one time*," he explained. "He may clear a profit of $2 or $3 by the time his expenses are paid." Then he hit me with the whammy. "The guys who *clean* the shirts and pants, though, get paid $2 or $3 *every single time* the shirt gets cleaned. A man will buy a shirt once, but he'll get it laundered dozens of times…"

It's true. And it shows you that selling things that are enjoyed (shirts) is good. Selling services that must be performed again and again (cleaning shirts) or selling items that are consumed (like sodas, for instance) is *even better*.

My oldest son, Noah, runs a vending machine business. He has three machines. I helped him start the business when he was six, taking a few road trips to pick up some items we found on eBay. Here's what's great about his vending machines. First, **the items he sells are consumable.** He's selling what goes in the machines- the drinks. People buy those all the time. They consume them, then buy another one. Sometimes they do this multiple times in the same day from the same machine.

Second, **the machines work for him when he's not there.** When I was cutting grass, I had to show up. No work, no pay. Noah, on the other hand, fills the machines once a week. He returns a week later to refill them and collect the money he made while he was at home playing with Legos, jumping on his trampoline, and doing his math lessons.

Third, **the process is so simple that almost anyone can do it.** I don't mean to be disrespectful to my little buddy, but what he's doing is just not that difficult of a business model to put together. Anyone else can be trained, including his younger brothers coming behind him, to do the same thing he's done with a virtual guarantee of similar success.

That's what I think you need in a business opportunity to truly set yourself to be financially independent. Opportunities that create residual income are the absolute best- the money that shows up again and again. The opportunity with Young Living is similar to Noah's vending business. The vending machines will work on his behalf while he's away, but *he has to continue filling them at regular intervals or the business dries up*.

We feel that multilevel marketing companies, and Young Living in particular, has provided an incredible opportunity for us to invest in something (a very minimal financial investment at that!) that will continue to grow over time. And while it does require some continual

> Selling services that must be performed again and again (cleaning shirts) or selling items that are consumed (like sodas, for instance) is *even better*.

maintenance, refilling and strategizing, it *doesn't* require a 40 hour work week to keep moving in the right direction. Because Young Living is set-up with a focus on team building, the more support we provide for our team, the more successful our team becomes and in turn the more successful we become. And it's better than filling your own machines by yourself.

And that, my friends, is a great reason to get comfortable with network marketing.

The dark side- Ponzi or Pyramid or. . .?

Yes, there *can* be a dark side of multilevel marketing. I read *The Four Year Career* on our plane *rides* back from Hawaii. Since we had a few connections to make, I decided to make the most of it. The author writes,

> *I have seen our profession dirty its pants with its own greed, selfishness, immaturity, and general lack of character within its leaders. I have heard all the rational experiences and factoids about how and why this profession is the scourge of the earth. Many of those perspectives are right on, well deserved and make total sense...*[174]

---

[174] *The Four Year Career*, Kindle Version, location 27.

Yes, we need to acknowledge that some people have been cheated, some people have been scammed, others have been pressured, and some have felt like they basically got lied to and every other kind of violation that can take place. You, or people you know, may even have a stash of stuff in your basement or garage that you *had to buy* in order to make the home-based business work. Many of the people we've met through Young Living, who are running extremely profitable essential oil businesses, now, were once in that same camp.

But they've found something that works with Young Living. Almost always, it's because they fell in love with product, the company, it's founders and staff- and then got comfortable with the idea that MLMs can work and still leave good relationships in tact. The author of *The Four Year Career* eventually determined this to be true for himself. He continues,

> *I have also seen that, for those who 'figure it out,' their lives are forever enriched financially, physically, emotionally, and spiritually. Some would say that those who succeed in Network Marketing is 'not fair.' I would say that anyone who 'takes a look' at Network Marketing as a part-time income or a significant wealth building alternative has the same opportunity to succeed.[175]*

Yes, **there can be a "dark side" of virtually everything. If something can be abused or misused, at some point somebody might likely figure out how to do it.** But that can't be the grid by which I make decisions. And I've decided that network marketing isn't inherently bad, either, just because someone has abused it before.

In my short time around the business, I have heard two chief arguments against Young Living:

- Arguments that center around slander concerning Gary Young

- Arguments that center around Ponzi schemes and Pyramid schemes

I shared my views and experiences concerning Gary in Chapter 1. Now, let me deal with the arguments that center around multilevel marketing specifically, the Ponzi and Pyramid arguments.

First, let's talk Ponzi, because Ponzi and Pyramid are really two different things. I did some checking online and found this: "A Ponzi scheme is a fraudulent investment operation where the operator, an individual or

---

[175] *The Four Year Career*, Kindle Version, location 27.

organization, pays returns to its investors from new capital paid to the operators by new investors, rather than from profit earned by the operator."[176]

Basically, what happens is simple to understand once you create a "real world example" to help you visualize it. Let's say that I'm at the top of the Ponzi, that I'm the one leading the scam and that I get you to invest. Here's what happens:

- I tell you that I'm investing in something- let's say it's beach front property in Dallas, Texas.

- You agree to invest because you think that Dallas is a booming town and that the new beach front condos will do well. I'm so persuasive that it never dawns on you that the nearest beach is several hundred miles away. In fact, I don't really give you much time to check into it, because it's a "now or never" opportunity I'm presenting to you. You agree to invest $100,000 with me- and I agree to pay you 20% per year- $20,000 at the end of 365 days. I may even agree to pay you that amount sooner if the business does well.

- I need to pay you a return on the investment. The problem is… well… there's no beachfront property in Dallas for me to develop. So, in order to get the money to pay you I find *another* investor. I sell him on the idea of the beachfront property. I offer him a good return, too, as long as he "acts now." I may even offer him a better rate than I offered you, because the deal gets harder and harder to sell as time goes on. People start wising up. Anyway, he gives me $100,000 as in investment.

> I've decided that network marketing isn't inherently bad, either, just because someone has abused it before.

- I go back to you and give you the $20,000 I agreed to give you, leaving me the original gain of $100,000 off you and $80,000 off him.

- Or, I show you the check and get you to reinvest it *back* into the Ponzi that I'm running. After all, you can't get a return like that anywhere else.

Most Ponzi schemes promise outrageous earnings, such as the example I used above. Why do people go for it? Because a skilled salesman sells them a pipe

---

[176] http://en.wikipedia.org/wiki/Ponzi_scheme, accessed 03-25-2014.

dream that, in their minds, is too good *not* to be true. And, the salesman pays them just enough to verify that it is, in fact, true. True on paper, at least.

Eventually the entire Ponzi collapses because the ringleader at the top runs out of people to scam. He finds it difficult to make the large payments back to the people who invested since, really, there were no goods or services ever being offered. It was just a false business plan and a bunch of numbers. By the way, this con-man game was named after Charles Ponzi, a guy who lived in 1920s Boston and was apparently incredibly skilled at selling people things that didn't exist.

Is Young Living a Ponzi? Clearly not, because…

- No set incomes are being promised.

- Actual goods are being sold. You can't go see my beachfront development in Dallas, but you can go walk the farms in Idaho or rummage through the warehouse in Salt Lake City. You can also pick up the oils, smell them, diffuse them, etc.

- There are no new investors needed to keep the machine going- people who enroll become distributors and immediately receive the goods when they are shipped to their homes.

- At the end of the day, the distributors have simply bought some items- whether they choose to use them or do anything else with them is up to them completely.

Second, you've probably been warned by now that Young Living is a Pyramid. Let me give you the official language of what a Pyramid is and then we'll discuss whether or not this is true about Young Living. Wikipedia states that "a pyramid scheme is an unsustainable business model that involves promising participants payment or services, primarily for enrolling other people into the scheme, rather than supplying any real investment or sale of products or services to the public."[177]

Notice that the Pyramid is different than the Ponzi in that the Pyramid deals with goods and services in a more tangible way. In a Pyramid the distributors may have lots of items on hand- all to lure others into the Pyramid. Keep in mind, the people in the Pyramid *probably don't know that they are in a scheme*- they're genuinely trying to enroll people into this great thing that they've found!

------

[177] http://en.wikipedia.org/wiki/Pyramid_scheme, accessed 03-25-2014.

Here's the hitch, though. In a Pyramid, the goods or services are not necessarily central to the entire operation- the enrollments are. The participants are paid primarily for enrolling people, not primarily for moving the goods through the distribution channels- even though there are lots of products sitting around.

As well, Pyramids always *aggressively* recruit new distributors- because that's how people "up the Pyramid" are getting paid. As such, they also offer "now or never" scenarios. They promise to give new enrollees huge payoffs in the future (usually sooner than later) in order to lure them in. Remember, the products are not as important as getting people to pay you to sign up.

Here's why you may feel a lot of pressure in a Pyramid situation: "In a Ponzi scheme, the schemer acts as a "hub" for the victims, interacting with all of them directly. In a pyramid scheme, those who recruit additional participants benefit directly."[178] In other words, in the Ponzi scheme there is one single man at the top that is usually benefitting. He wants to keep things on the "down low," because the more people that hear about the investment opportunity the more he runs a risk of being exposed. In a Pyramid, people aren't concerned about exposure- they want hype, lots of it. They want people to think that everyone *is* enrolling so that more people *will* enroll. They are paid from those enrollments.

When the "shine" dulls (or disappears) the schemes are usually revealed for what they are- get rich quick opportunities. The products are usually of an inferior quality. Remember, the Pyramid wasn't about the products anyway. It was

> Everyone can find a network marketing / pyramid scheme / multilevel marketing horror story if they want to.

about the "sign ups." In time, everyone discovers that they were just putting lipstick on a pig or polishing a poop. The hype dies and people move on.

Now, granted, a distributor in Young Living may pressure you. Or, they may genuinely be excited about the oils and you may *feel* like they're pressuring you- even if that's not their intent. At the end of the day, though, once you understand the commission structure for Young Living, you'll see that it's clearly not a Pyramid.[179]

---

[178] http://en.wikipedia.org/wiki/Ponzi_scheme#Unraveling_of_a_Ponzi_scheme, accessed 03-25-2014.

[179] See *The Husband's Guide to the Comp Plan* for more info on this.

When I was in Hawaii, I heard stories over and over of successful distributors who had changed their up-line or stayed dormant for *years* because someone above them was pressuring them to perform. Someone above them created a Pyramid culture, even though Young Living is not a pyramid. Think about that: Someone above them could have *benefited* from their labor sooner had they just "been chill" with the whole thing.[180]

Here's the deal: **a high pressure situation is not good for anyone. It's not fun and it makes you feel bad when things don't work out in the way you planned.** Plus, you want to leave the door open for those who say "No" to come back to you later on. If you pressure them and they feel like they've let you

> ... there are industry standards that govern how multilevel marketing companies must operate. You can check these against any opportunity you see and determine on your own if the company is legit.

down, they won't likely feel like they can come back. Be gracious and always leave the door open- even when they say no.[181]

By the way, there are industry standards that govern how multilevel marketing companies must operate. You can check these against any opportunity you see and determine on your own if the company is legit.

For the company to operate legally and ethically, it must do each of the following[182]:

- Sell viable products at a market price as its main objective

- Not promise potential incomes to potential members- or even infer them without the appropriate legal jargon[183]

---

[180] The flip side, though, is that the person who eventually became successful could have become successful much sooner, too, and benefited themselves.

[181] It may be a "No, for now, but not for later" situation- even if they don't have words to articulate it- or even know so themselves. I'll talk more about this concept in a future chapter.

[182] See *The Four Year Career*, Kindle location 148f.

[183] This is one of the reasons you will see Young Living refuse to create spreadsheets of potential income. As well, you will often see corporate remind distributors that they cannot offer certain types of incentives for enrollments. They do this to keep everyone in the bounds of "fair play" and keep things above board.

- Not pay recruiting fees- income must be derived totally from the sale of the products

Young Living is good on all counts. The products are the focus, no incomes are promised, and you aren't offered any recruiting fees.

Every one can find a network marketing / pyramid scheme / multilevel marketing horror story if they want to. Heck, you can find a Wal-Mart horror story, too. Don't let someone's train wreck of an experience derail you from something that might be helpful to your future. Study it for yourself and do what you think is best.

That said, here's a chart comparing Young Living with a Pyramid scheme:

Pyramid scheme vs. Young Living

Pyramid scheme	Young Living
Requires a significant investment up front	The max investment is $150, for which you receive a diffuser and 11 oils
Pressure to "sign now" or "miss out forever"	You can sign up whenever you want to- and enroll under anyone
Promises you significant financial return	No financial gain is promised, though the commission structure is provided to you if you choose to work the business side- a relatively small percentage of distributors ever elect to work the business side
Focuses on money, not goods or services	The products are the focus
Difficult to get good information	All information is readily available, regarding the products as well as financial opportunities
Fizzles and is exposed as an empty promise in due time (usually rather quickly)	Young Living has been around for 20 years- and is growing (their best month to date was the month in which I began writing this book, March 2014)

More people buying less = more

Now that we know how things shouldn't work in a legitimate multilevel marketing company, let's see if we can shed some light on how things *should* work. First, you need to understand that there's a profound difference between traditional sales models (i.e., big box stores, small storefronts alike, and online purchases alike) and network marketing sales models.

In a network marketing model, no single person sells a lot of products. Sure, a few exceptions may exist, but **most people who are successful spend their time building a large team with a lot of people who will all do a little bit**- not a small team of a few people who will do a lot. Read that sentence again. See if it makes sense. After studying the Young Living compensation plan, it seems obvious to me that the way to make more money over the long haul is to go the first route above and build a bigger team, not build a small team of a few people buying a lot of products.

Think about it: if your income is tied to how much you sell, then your income is tied to your efforts, to your own output. In effect, you simply own another job. If you don't perform, you don't get paid. You're back to cutting the grass, again.

> ... there's a profound difference between traditional sales models (i.e., big box stores, small storefronts alike, and online purchases alike) and network marketing sales models.

If, on the other hand, your income is tied to the efforts of an entire team of people, then your income is more stable. If one person quits, you don't sink the ship. In fact, if you're building your team right, there's probably two or three more distributors coming right behind them.[184]

Other differences between traditional sales models and network marketing models include the amount of time people are required to work (if you have a sales job your boss is probably going to demand that you're there full time- or you'll be fired), as well as how you are paid (in a true sales job you'll have a quota or you'll work on commission).

By contrast, MLMs allow you to choose *when* and *how much* you work. As well, instead of being tied to a specific territory, you're allowed to work anywhere

---

[184] I'll share with you in my writing on the compensation plan, too, why you really shouldn't sell kits and large amounts of other items to people- why, instead, you should enroll them as a distributor and teach them how to purchase their own. The short version is that 1) it's a better financial deal for them- and for you, and 2) it gives them the opportunity of earning a future income if they choose to work the "business side" at some point.

without limits. And, instead of having a quota, you'll be rewarded with incentives. The chart below highlights some of these differences.[185]

The first and last points in the chart are interesting. In a typical sales force, you might have 100 sales people trying to move $100,000 worth of products in a year to net $10,000,000 worth of sales for the company. In a network marketing scenario- or, let's just say it, a multilevel organization- you may have 10,000 people moving $1,000 in that year to achieve that same $10,000,000 mark.[186]

In this way, more people are buying less (or even selling less) to create the same revenue stream). **It's the difference between a lot of people doing a little bit as opposed to a few people doing a lot.**

Compare & Contrast- Sales vs. Network Marketing

Sales	Network marketing
A few people do a lot	A lot of people each do a little
Work full time	Work "some" time
Sales people	Distributors
Employees	Distributors
Quota	Incentive
Protected and / or limited territory	Go anywhere
Generate more volume yourself	Generate less volume yourself, more with a team

So how do some people make such massive sums of money in MLM scenarios? Well, you have to remember that the company doesn't have the high overhead that other businesses have. They don't pay rent for multiple storefronts, they don't pay utility bills on those storefronts, and they don't have massive payroll expenses. Sure, they have overhead expenses at the corporate offices, but every business has these. That leaves the corporation with the ability to invest

---

[185] This chart is adapted from *The Four Year Career*. See Kindle version, location 339.

[186] I learned this contrast from *The Four Year Career*, Kindle location 339.

all of those dollars in their distribution channels, which happen to be their people.

Lessons from the thrift store

I told you a bit about the ministry I lead, The Village, in the intro chapter.[187] Currently, it takes about $1,000,000 annually to run the organization (which will increase with the costs of running the store). Of that million, I have to raise about $30,000 a month in order to keep things moving forward. Some months I hit it, some months I don't. During those times, we just hang on and hope that we had a great previous month or an extra-good next month. It seems to always work out.

Our business manager and I decided we needed to create an income stream that would alleviate that stress-creating $30,000 gap each month. We needed a massive vending machine, in other words, that we could stock and then collect money from. Enter our newest project, The Village Thrift.[188]

For about a year we studied various models, interviewed several people who were running actual stores and were willing to share their experience with us, and decided this would be a great course of action. If we can move the store to generating $80,000 in sales per month, it will remove the fundraising pressure we feel each month.

So far, the experience has been incredible. The Lord sent an incredible leader to oversee the operation (probably one of the top ten qualified guys *in the nation*). We found a 45,000 square foot facility less than two miles from our current ministry center at what is reported to be the busiest intersection in West Birmingham. The landlord was willing to give us six months rent-free in order to get the thing up and running. We'll have the thing open by the time this book goes to print and we'll know if the whole thing worked.

To show you the difference in this type of business model vs. the multilevel marketing model, I'll highlight eight basics about the store- from a business perspective. I'm going to walk you through them, and then compare and contrast with what happened when Cristy began cranking up her home-based

---

[187] www.WelcomeToTheVillage.net

[188] www.TheVillageThrift.net

Young Living business. I think looking at these two side-by-side will be quite revealing to you.

First, we've had to invest a lot of money to even get the doors open at the thrift store- before we know if the store will be successful or not. I think we'll succeed fantastically, but at the end of the day *I really don't know*. I'm taking one big educated guess. Ray, the guy who came onboard to lead the store, has almost 30 years of experience in thrift stores. He told me we would need $100,000 to open the doors.

"We don't have that much," I told him. "Let's try to do it for $50,000."

So far, we've landed somewhere around $60,000- an incredibly low number for opening a store the size we are opening. And that's with getting stellar deals on lots of items. For instance, we bought out three Bama Fever stores and took all of their check out counters, their racks, and every hangar and bag they had- plus mannequins and fixtures and computers- for $2,000. Ray negotiated and bought every shelf and counter from a closed-down Movie Gallery for $300. We found ways to build expensive racks ourselves and save about $8,000 instead of purchasing them for $15,000. Another organization donated $10,000 worth of wood. Ray's number is closer to what we would have spent without all of these factors. So we got a great deal- but we still spent a lot of money before even opening the doors.

Second, we've had to find inventory. Specifically, we've had to find 80,000 items of clothing, 10,000 pairs of shoes, 5,000 toys, 200 pieces of furniture, and thousands of other assorted items just to fill the sales floor. Then, we've had to find virtually that same number again in order to fill the stock room, so that we don't run out of merchandise the first week we open the store. We'll have to keep the stock flowing to keep the doors open.

Ray assured me that if we placed a few donation drop boxes around town, and if we got the word out, people would start dropping off their used stuff. So we built 15 boxes,

> ... we still spent a lot of money before even opening the doors.

painted them yellow, and started tossing them in parking lots in high traffic areas. I soon learned that Ray had *under-stated* his case. The goods started coming in faster than I ever thought possible. I got excited, bought some more wood, and put the guys to constructing 10 more!

Our model, of course, is different than a "real store." We don't look online and search through catalogs and order things we think people want. We simply take what people give- *and we take it for free*. Our inventory costs are dramatically lower, then, than a department store of the same size. However, we still have to manage truck schedules, repair broken drop boxes, and keep the inventory coming. If we don't go pick it up, we don't get it. That's reality.

Third, we're dealing with payroll on an entirely new level. When I started the ministry, I made payroll easy. There were only two of us- me and another guy.

"I'll pay you once a month," I told him. "The final day of the month I'll pay you your salary for that entire month."

He agreed, so that's the way I paid myself and him from then on. I figured that you pay the power bill once a month and you pay the rent or mortgage once a month, so just pay the people once a month, give them a big check, and let them manage it all month instead of in two week increments or whatever time frame it is when most people get paid.

We never changed that system- *until now*. Yes, everyone on staff at the ministry is either on salary or they are interns and receive a stipend. But the thrift store has opened our world to an entirely new dimension- the hourly employee who gets paid every single week and works a slightly different number of hours each week. This means you can't just look at payroll from 30 days ago, see what it was, and duplicate it. It means you have to actually do *more* work.

Fourth, we now have more facilities to manage. Our ministry center is open 24 hours a day and houses up to 150 people at a time. We clean the entire thing twice a day, replace at least *some* light bulbs daily, and constantly repair broken toilets and sinks. We've painted the entire thing twice in two years. It's just the way it is when you have that many people living in one place.

I thought we were property pros, but the thrift store has taken everything to an entirely new level. In order to open the thrift store, we had to remove 24,000 square feet of tile, purchase over 100 gallons of paint, buy 13,000 pounds of angle iron, and locate over 500 utility wheels for production carts. That's an absurd amount of stuff to do- and that's only a *small* fraction of the bigger equation.

You can't just walk in and start selling stuff, either. You have to prep the facilities, call the inspectors, make sure you have fire extinguishers, and make everybody in the shopping center around you happy. You need a business license for that location. *Then* you can open. If you have any energy left. And money. You still need money to operate.

Fifth, I'm now advertising and blogging and looking to get the word out about the project. Sure, it's been fun- and now a whole lot more people have heard about our ministry that would never have heard about it before seeing a yellow drop box, making a clothing donation, or going online out of curiosity. In order to make this happen, though, we've had to create and order signage (it looks fabulous, by the way!), and create a whole "look and feel" for what we're doing. I shoot a new video each week. That's more time, more energy… and, yes… more cash.

Sixth, now there's more work to do, more hours in the week. The new business is not going to simply run itself. That store will be open at least 10 hours each day, 6 days a week. As well, we think there's probably 20 more hours of stuff to do just to manage things.

I can either work these hours- or I can pay someone else to work them. I can't be everywhere at once, and I can't work 80 more hours per week above what I'm already working. Nor can I do the work of 8 or 10 people at once, so we've hired more people. That's more to manage, more to pay for, and more that could potentially go wrong. At this point, it's all going smoothly… but you get the point. Opening a business is complex and gets more exponentially complex the deeper you get into it.

Seventh, the learning curve is steep- and it comes *fast*. Everything I thought I knew about thrift stores- even after studying them for a year from reputable sources- has proven mostly wrong when I finally got into the trenches.

Ray knows thrift stores so well that he can tell you how many items of clothing are in a full drop box. He can tell you how many unusable items will be in there that people decided to dump on us instead of just tossing in the trash. He can tell you how much money that box will convert to once you get those good items on the floor. He can tell you that the average customer will spend $11.35 when they enter the store, so you need about 280 customers a day to hit just over $3,000 in sales a day to hit $80,000 each month.

> Opening a business is complex and gets more exponentially complex the deeper you get into it.

I can regurgitate that now on paper, but I'm not sure exactly how it works. I'm not even clear how the stuff gets from the box where you donate to our truck to the storage containers on site to the production area and then to the sales floor. I'm still learning- and I'm learning fast. You have to when you have a business.

Eighth, finally, we have a great deal of financial exposure if the thing fails. In fact, if it fails, it will probably sink the ministry. We've invested money into the store for the short term that we think will make us financially stronger in the long term. That money could have been used to run the ministry for a few months, though.

I remember sitting in a board meeting when I told the directors how much cash we had on hand. The consensus was unanimous.

"Push all the chips to the center of the table," one of the men said.

Then another- "Focus hard and get the store open quick."

The truth is the time we've invested in setting the store into motion could have been used to do actual ministry. That's the trade off. We were willing to make the trades, though, because we believe that in the long turn (as in not too long from now) the store will free us up financially and time-wise. We won't have to spend as much time chasing donations- we'll be generating our own. And our financial health won't be as dependent upon *me* raising the money, it will be dependent on an entire team's efforts to run a profitable store that has extremely low overhead and an amazingly high profit margin.

Is there an easier way?

Here's the reason I went into all of that detail for you: Cristy didn't start her Young Living business with $60,000- or whatever the number will finally be by the time we open the doors. She paid $150 and received products worth that much.

If the start-up for a home-based business was more than that, we probably wouldn't have been able to do it. Ever. But, because of the relatively low cost of getting started, she was in at a low price. **And she was buying healthy products that make us healthier, items that we would have used anyway**. And she was buying them not thinking that she would ever do a business- *anything* with Young Living.

Yes, *now* she invests money back into the business each month. We currently set aside $1,000 from each check to re-invest. She is able to buy educational and promotional materials, she offers monthly incentives to her team, and she gives away products to people who might benefit from them. She also pays for our family's stash of oils and other Young Living supplies with this money.

However, **she never had to put money into the business until the business was giving her money first.**

Cristy doesn't have to deal with inventory, either- not like we do at the thrift store. People order straight from Young Living. If she teaches a class and people enroll, they pay Young Living and the company ships the new items directly to them. Cristy can always look online to see how her business is doing, but she doesn't have to manage the numbers and send out the items. Young Living handles it all.

She doesn't even create promotional materials. She "advertises," if you consider posting testimonials and talking about the oils. But she's not had to create a "brand" like we have had to do with our thrift store. Because of the support of her upline and the Lemon Dropper team she is on, that's all handled. In addition, she recently uploaded a "plug in and play" website she bought for a low nominal fee from a third-party supplier.

She doesn't manage payroll, either- not even for herself. Often, in a small business or home-based business the owner of the company pays all of the bills and then pays themselves *if there is money left.* This means that sometimes the owner doesn't get paid. I've heard of some MLMs where the distributor collects all of the money and then sends in what's not theirs, keeping what would be the equivalent of their incentive pay for the month. Either scenario requires some sort of accounting and keeping up with the things that you track. Mess up, and you could lose big.

> Cristy didn't start her Young Living business with $60,000- or whatever the number will finally be by the time we open the doors. She paid $150 and received products worth that much.

Yes, Cristy places an order each month. Many times friends and family will order something on that order- meaning they owe her a few dollars for an item. But that is simple compared to anything I've mentioned above.

Cristy doesn't manage facilities for the business- other than the upstairs room that has been reconfigured to make a small office space. We were already paying the utilities for that room with our monthly power and water bill, so everything's covered. No new expenses like the massive bill I'm getting for the thrift store.

And, sure, there has been a bit of a learning curve, but we're learning as we go. She's been using natural and herbal remedies for a decade, so she's not into new territory.

One of the greatest blessings, though, is that our family never really had any financial exposure if the thing failed. We didn't invest much to get in, so we didn't tie up money that needed to go elsewhere. At the end of the day, even if we were going to jump into it for the business side only, it would have been a safe gamble.

Here's a cheat sheet to illustrate what I just told you. Notice the differences here:

The Village Thrift vs. Cristy's Young Living Business

	Thrift store	Young Living
Start-up capital required	$60,000 and growing- even with all the deals we got	$150
Inventory	Yes	No
Inventory management	Yes	As much / little as you want
Payroll- manage it?	Yes	No
Buildings	Yes	Run it from our house
Utilities	Yes	Already paid for when we pay for our house
Advertising	Some	As much / little as you want
Liability insurance	Yes	No
Hours required / week	Staff covering 80-plus hours / week	You decide
Learning curve	Steep and comes fast	Learn as you go, at your own pace
Financial exposure if you fail	Yes- major loss- and you lose money and time that could have been invested somewhere else	None- you spent $150 on products you would have likely bought anyway

More about who gets paid

Network marketing works best when you're selling something you would buy anyway- something you would purchase even if you weren't attached to a network marketing group. Young Living is *perfect* for us. Remember, we were using oils and natural remedies, anyway. Cristy wasn't seeking a business opportunity, she only needed a night away from the house. She enrolled simply to get the oils, hoping she could sell enough to pay for her own.

You might be surprised that most people who are involved with a multilevel marketing company don't maintain their relationship with the company for the paycheck. They do it to become customers, because they genuinely like the products they're receiving. According to *The Four Year Career*, for every company, you have the following categories of distributors:[189]

- **Customers**. These members buy the monthly minimums (if required) or less. Many of them initially try the business side and decide it's not for them. They love the products and continue using them, though.

- **Retailers**. These members typically sell only enough to "fund their habit." They are content to do this, as they love the products and would have been using them anyway. If they can do a little work and get theirs for free, even better.

- **Network marketers**. These are the people who aggressively work the business side. They understand the income potential and work the system, making

> ... most people who are involved with a multilevel marketing company don't maintain their relationship with the company for the paycheck.

thousands to tens of thousands per month. Ironically, some of these people- in fact, most of them- started as customers and then found themselves making money. At that point, they decided to pursue the possibility.

The Four Year Career suggest that "Most network marketing distributors start out pursuing the income opportunity, but once they give up they settle into being a customer. Most companies' total sales are made of these 'wholesale customers.' Maybe they sell enough to 'get theirs for free.' This is easily 90% of

---

[189] This information comes from *The Four Year Career*, Kindle version, location 298.

most network marketing sales forces. The other 10% is made up of those earning a few hundred a month. Less than 1% build a sales force of these users and sellers such that they qualify for the 'four year career.'"[190]

How does Young Living compare with other MLMs?

	Typical multilevel	Young Living
Customer	90%	85%
Retailer	10%	10%
Network marketing	1%	5%

A quick observation here: as I've told you a few times in this book, I've yet to meet anyone who jumped into Young Living for a money-making opportunity, as *The Four Year Career* suggests. I'm sure they exist- and, if they do, it's a legitimate and honorable way to seek a job (to go find a MLM and enroll).

In fact, *The Four Year Career* argues that you should do just that- go find a reputable MLM and join it. Then commit to working it for four years somewhat aggressively. At that point, you will reach critical mass and you will be able to coast, possibly even retiring from your current job. Hence, the title *The Four Year Career.* The point of that book is that if you can actually create a "pyramid" (there's the nasty word, I know, but they use it in a good way).

Other books I read while researching to write this *Field Guide* said there are three groups in network marketing organizations:

1. Simply buy the product

2. Sell enough to buy their own for free

3. Aggressively work the business

You'll notice that those categories are similar to what I found in *The Four Year Career.*

James and Stacy McDonald are a ministry couple that have been involved with the business side of Young Living for about three years. James is a pastor in

---

[190] Kindle location 164.

Central Illinois, where he and Stacy have ten children.[191] Four of the kids are grown and married, giving them five grandchildren. The wedding for another is being planned as I write. I first met James about 6 years ago at a homeschool convention in my hometown of Birmingham, where he was one of the keynote speakers.

We bumped into James and Stacy on the Hawaii trip. There, James gave me some advice about Young Living. We passed him and his wife, Stacy, walking outside at the hotel the final evening. I knew they had become successful in the business and asked how long they had been at it. In a sense, it would give me some benchmarks to expect in terms of time and commitment, particularly as I was starting to think about charting some goals and a plan to make this work in light of Cristy's initial success.

"Have you read *The Four Year Career*?" he asked.

I hadn't. In fact, I hadn't even heard of the book. I nodded as such. James is the reason I went and downloaded the book on my Kindle app and began reading it the following day.

> ... he was painting the picture of what I had been thinking all along- at some point you pick up momentum. and it becomes much easier.

"The author talks about pushing a car uphill," James continued. "Up a very slight, rolling hill." He moved his hand like a cresting wave. "At some point that car levels and becomes easier to push... Then," he offered as he swooped his hand towards the ground, "the car simply rolls on its own. You don't push anymore at that point- you just jump in and ride."[192]

James wasn't suggesting that we simply work the business side of Young Living, push it hard for a few years, and then quit. Rather, he was painting the picture of what I had been thinking all along- at some point you pick up momentum and it becomes much easier.

Young Living is a global company whose marketing strategy is to succeed through your success.

- They don't open retail stores, they distribute through your house.

---

[191] http://www.providencecpc.org/

[192] See *The Four Year Career*, Chapter 8, "Momentum," Kindle Version, location 509. It was after speaking to James that night than I went and ordered the book through Amazon and had it delivered to my iPad for $2.99.

- They don't pay a bazillion of executives, they pay you.

- They don't have an expensive marketing budget (though they put out some great materials), they pay you to market for them.

However, you have to decide which role you want in the company. Because it's a legitimate multilevel, YL is not going to promise you large checks for becoming a business builder.[193] You have to make the determination of what you want to do-whether you want to be a member who may occasionally enroll someone but primarily just wants great products, whether you want to enroll and sell enough to pay for your own, or whether you want to run a business that could be significantly lucrative for you and your future.

After talking to James, I read *The Four Year Career* and noticed that the following business model was promoted by its author:

- You enroll, and your organization has 1 business builder.

- You enroll 4 business builders directly under you / organization now has 5 business builders (to have 4 business builders, you will most likely enroll 16 or more people). This happens in year 1.

- They enroll 4 business builders each / organization now has the original 5 plus this level of 16 (4 people enrolling 4 each), for a total of 21 business builders. This happens in year 2.

- Those 16 also enroll 4 more (16 x 4 = 64), so now 75 business builders exist... all happening in year 3.

- Your level 4 grows to 256 deep (all 64 enroll 4 each = 64 x 4 = 256), so now 331 business builders exist. This happens in year 4.

The book suggests you can do this in four years *if you work hard.* You'll then be in that 1% that achieve success. As well, most people who earn money in a MLM don't make hundreds of thousands of dollars each year. "While earning potential varies by company and sales ability... the median *annual* income for those in direct sales is $2,400."[194]

---

[193] In April 2014 Young Living released a document titled "2013 U.S. Income Disclosure Statement," which shows the average incomes- and hours worked- for people at every distributor level in the organization.

[194] Peterecca, Laura (September 14, 2009). "What kind of business do you want to start?". *USAToday* (Gannett Company). pp. 4B. Emphasis added.

I've seen people in Young Living build strong organizations with relative ease, compared to what *The Four Year Career* proposes. And I've watched people on our team consistently break that financial threshold, to where they earn the average median income on a monthly basis.

The premise of *The Four Year Career* is that a strong leader may have 100 or so people in their organization at some point in the third year. Cristy had that many people on her team in a few months- as do people in her organization, now. And, there are people we know- the wives of some of the men who penned testimonials for this book- who built organizations much quicker.

Whatever the case, the scenario painted by *The Four Year Career* is far more appealing than the life plan many of us unknowingly settled into before coming onboard as distributors with Young Living:

- 40 hours of work per week

- 40 years of those work weeks

- 40% of the paycheck you earned is the amount you will live off during retirement[195]

In one of my interactions with Travis Ogden, the COO at Young Living, I learned that Young Living has about 300,000 active distributors, though the number of total members is well over one million at this point. He estimated the following:

- 85% just get in to buy the oils [these are our "customers" in the scenarios I've presented above].

- 10% sell enough to "fund their habit" [these are our "retailers," by way of comparison].

- 5% create a profitable business [these are our "network marketers"].[196]

His estimates jive with the *2013 U.S. Income Disclosure Statement* released by Young Living in April 2014: 92% of all members are ranked as Distributors; 8% are ranked as Star (the lowest level for an active business builder) or above.

---

[195] See *The Four Year Career*, Kindle location 75, for a more thorough description.

[196] FaceBook private message, March 4, 2014.

Only 1% of all distributors are at the "Gold" level, where the average income last year was $6,527/month- $78,324/year.[197]

Those numbers are indicative of a truly healthy organization- and not a Ponzi or Pyramid scheme. Remember, in those schemes people are simply part of the organization to make money- not use the products. As such, a Pyramid will have numbers that are almost the opposite of Young Living's. I'd expect to see 85-90% or more working the business in a Pyramid.

Clearly, most people go to Young Living for the products- not the profit potential. And, the company is currently in it's 20th year. The company grew 8-12% each year for the first 18 years. Last year, business boomed- the company grew by 35%.[198] In some divisions growth actually topped 100%. Remember, though, the company is 20 years old. Pyramids die quickly once the sizzle settles. They don't grow steadily over time and gain momentum like Young Living is doing.

Some people go looking for a network marketing / MLM- and I suppose that's ok. We didn't do that. We tried the oils, loved them and it was natural for us to talk about them. We weren't told we would "get rich quick" by our upline- or by anyone else for that matter. But as we shared our story, how the oils blessed our family, we were rewarded for sharing the product with others. That's a good thing.

It is saturated?

One of my co-workers suggested the Young Living market might be saturated, that he and his wife probably wouldn't become distributors because there was no one left to sign up. Market saturation wasn't a concern for us when Cristy enrolled. Again, she got

> ... the company is 20 years old. Pyramids die quickly once the sizzle settles. They don't grow steadily over time and gain momentum like Young Living is doing.

---

[197] Young Living released a document titled "2013 U.S. Income Disclosure Statement," which shows the average incomes- and hours worked- for people at every distributor level in the organization. It does not promise incomes- it simply relays what people at various levels throughout the organization made. And, it reveals the percentage of distributors at each rank.

[198] Stats provided by Travis Ogden.

in "just to buy our own." Then she hoped to sell enough to pay for ours. Honestly, if you're thinking about market saturation, you're looking at things like a Pyramid- where the income is driving the opportunity rather than the product.

"We'll just buy the oils from you when we need them," my co-worker said. Then he repeated his line, "The market is saturated now."

I told him two things.

First, even if you don't want to work the business side, it's a better deal for you to sign up as a distributor, anyway. Remember, most people involved in networking marketing companies aren't aggressively working the business side. They're simply signing up to buy products, much in the same way that people are joining Costco and Sam's Club just to get a better deal on the merchandise they buy every week or so *anyway*. You don't have to make a purchase from Young Living every month in order to be a member- you only have to make a purchase if you're going to get a commission check.[199]

Second, the market is *not* saturated. Sure, it's mathematically *possible* that the market will get saturated at some point, but "history has proven that saturation is not an issue."[200] With 7 billion people alive in the world today, there are plenty of people who aren't yet reached.

Think about it like this. I know of several multilevel / network marketing companies. They include: Advocare, Amway, Arbonne, Avon, Herbalife, Mary Kay, Primerica, and Tupperware. That's just a few of them.

The truth is that you're probably not a distributor in any of those organizations- meaning the market is not saturated. My co-worker happens to be among the billions who have *not* signed up yet for any of these, too, including Young Living. He knows me well, and knows that YL paid for us to go to Hawaii. The saturation still hasn't yet soaked him, though!

In reality, you'd probably have to think long and hard to name more than two or three friends, co-workers, family members, or even acquaintances who are distributors *for any* of the other organizations I just named as well. And those are all really big, really successful companies- most of them larger than Young

---

[199] I'll talk more about this when we work through the compensation plan.

[200] *The Four Year Career*, Kindle Version, location 312.

Living. I didn't even know all of their names and had to Google to find most of them. Do you see what I'm saying? Saturation is really not the issue.[201]

The laborers who worked the field all day

There's a little known parable in the end of Matthew's Gospel. It's the parable of laborers in the field, and has become a new lenses through how I view Young Living and the opportunity before us.[202] The parable can seem classically confusing- like many of Jesus' teachings. Here's how it goes:

The owner of a vineyard went and gathered people who were eager to work one morning. Jesus says that the first wave of workers came early in the morning. In that culture, we would expect this to be at 6:00 am, the official start of the day.[203]

> Sure, it's mathematically possible that the market will get saturated at some point, but "history has proven that saturation is not an issue."

Apparently, the owner went to the nearby labor pool again around 9:00 am and hired more workers. As was the case with the first, he agreed to pay them a fair wage.[204] For some reason, the man continued going back and hiring more workers. He picked up a few more workers around noon, just as people would be taking a break for lunch.[205] Then he did the oddest thing of all- even odder than the getting more workers halfway through the day. He went again at 5:00

---

[201] *The Four Year Career* estimates that 475,000 people become involved in network marketing companies each year (Kindle Version, location 200). In the same time, 361,481 babies are born (source: ask.com, accessed 03/06/2014). In other words, the field is growing- but just slightly faster that population growth as a whole. There's still plenty of room to work the field.

[202] Matthew 20:1-16

[203] Their days started at 6pm at night. Night officially ran from 6pm until 6am. Then "day" began. It ran until 6pm, when the new day began. In other words, they rested first. Look at Genesis 1 and you'll notice that the Bible reads "there was evening and then morning, the first day…" Anyway, this means the 3rd hour of the day is 9am, the 6th hours is 12noon, the 9th hour is 3pm, etc… Conversely, the 6th hour of night would be 12pm.

[204] Matthew 20:3

[205] Matthew 20:5

pm, almost quitting time, and hired a few more. Again, he agreed that he would pay them whatever was fair.[206]

It makes you wonder why these guys weren't already working somewhere else. Were they lazy? Were they *not* there the first time the man picked up all of the other workers? Had they finished a first job, and were needing additional work/income? Or was he impressed that they were still there, hoping someone would hire them, so he finally sympathetically gave them a shot...? We don't know.

We do know that the closing bell rang around 6:00 pm, the end of the day, and the man began calling everyone in from their toil. He started passing out payroll *in reverse order* of how people were hired.[207]

This is when something even stranger than the man's odd hiring pattern happened:

- He paid those who had worked only an hour as if they had worked for a *full* day. They were ecstatic- they were paid more than 10 times the number of hours they had worked![208]

- He then paid those who arrived at lunch time as if they, too, had been there all day. They were likewise thrilled. They had been paid "double for their trouble."

- The payments continued with the men who arrived around 9:00 am. They had put in 9 hours. He paid them for 12, for a full day of work. They were pleased.

- Finally, he called the group that had started early in the morning... and he paid them... *the same amount that he had paid every other person.* They were frustrated- and shared their angst *openly*.

"Did you not agree to work for these wages?" the owner asked. "Did I mislead you or not pay you what was right...?"[209]

They couldn't argue. He had. They had been paid *exactly* what *they agreed* to work for.

---

[206] Matthew 20:6

[207] Matthew 20:8

[208] Remember, a typical day ran from 6am to 6pm. So a full day would have been 12 hours.

[209] Matthew 20:13

"I didn't give the others what belongs to you," he explained. "Why would you begrudge my generosity to someone else…?"[210]

I know, you're wondering… *What does this have to do with anything related to Young Living?*

Quite simply this: Cristy and I feel like the laborers who showed up late in the day. You might, too.

On one level, I want you to know that there's still room for you to turn this into a great business opportunity for your family. You can still get paid what everyone else gets paid. On another level, I want you to know that there are a ton of laborers who have been in the field for years and have been tilling the soil and making the field more workable for you. There are people who have been working in Young Living for years, a decade… even 15 or 20 years. They have figured out the system and created an environment in which we can succeed. We have been invited into their workplace, very late in the game. And, no, I don't think we're in the 11th hour of the day- I don't think it's anywhere close to "quitting time."

My hat goes off to all of those who have been working. Frankly, I don't know how they had the measure of success they've had without the use of FaceBook (which has exponentially grown my wife's business), cell phones, email on phones, and the less expensive and faster ways of creating marketing pieces that we use today. What did they do before the boom of the Internet? What did they do without the use of all of the tools we have? I consider the first Young Living distributors to be brilliant pioneers. They have paved the way for us to be successful. They've allowed us to join their party.

Rumor is that Mary Young was instrumental in changing the compensation plan not too long ago- for the purposes of helping people succeed in the business and jump rank (be encouraged) even faster. Think about the opportunity that is ahead of you. I heard that people are now moving through the ranks quicker than ever before. In my forthcoming discussion on the compensation plan, I'll coach you up to

> I want you to know that there's still room for you to turn this into a great business opportunity for your family. You can still get paid what everyone else gets paid.

---

[210] Matthew 20:14-15

Diamond.[211] There are higher ranks, but I think hitting Diamond could potentially enable you to become "financially free."

Here's the exciting part: it used to take years and years (even a decade!) to hit the Diamond mark. Then a strange thing happened. Alyssa shattered the previous record. She made it there in 18 months. I sent her a message to verify. She did- and told me her husband had just "retired."[212] After she broke the record, another person hit it in close to the same amount of time. Sharnael began working the business and became a Diamond- also around 18 months. Now she is free to minister and not worry about resources. And most recently, Monique shattered that record, hitting Diamond in 10 months! Why? Because she took hold of her opportunity to work in the "proverbial" field. Yes, she showed up later than the other workers, but there was still room for her (and you!) to work and be successful. The stage had been set by many previous laborers. When it was her turn, then she got in *and worked!*

> If you have a kit- or, more accurately if your wife does- you're already a distributor. Whether you do anything with it is up to you.

We've jumped in!

So here's where I am now: We're working the business side. And I'm encouraging you to consider it. I'm not selling you on it; I'm simply showing you what's possible with something you've already bought into. If you have a kit- or, more accurately if your wife does- you're already a distributor. Whether you do anything with it is up to you.

---

[211] *The Husband's Field Guide to the Comp Plan*

[212] I sent a message to Alyssa to verify this. She writes, "Yes, 18 months. Starting building in April of 2012 and hit it in October 2013. My husband retired last month" (FaceBook private message, March 25, 2014). This is simply awesome!

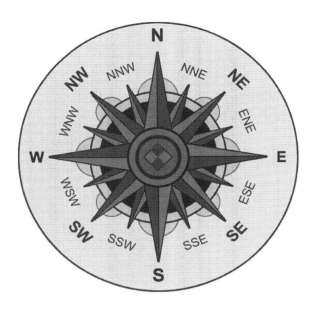

04: Direction: get comfortable with it

Action steps

☐ Get an answer, in your mind, for each of the following:

> **The main idea:** If you have a kit- or, more accurately if your wife does- you're already a distributor. Whether you do anything with it is up to you. Get comfortable with the possibilities…

☐ "It's multilevel marketing! Why would you do that?!?!"

☐ _____

☐ _____

☐ _____

☐ "It's too expensive to join! Is there another alternative?"[213]

☐ _____

☐ _____

☐ _____

☐ Here are a few reasons you might want to work the business side of Young Living- or any other multilevel marketing company:[214] Review each of these and see if they make sense for you and your family.

    ☐ Residual income, retirement, chained to the desk / saw / hammer / forklift / store

    ☐ Work from anywhere

    ☐ Low start-up costs (I$150)

    ☐ The comparative cost of an investment that will generate the same monthly residuals[215]

    ☐ You are in business *for* yourself but not in business *by* yourself

    ☐ You can "learn while you earn"

☐ Which of the above make the most sense to you, and meet the needs of your family?

---

[213] Note: you can become a distributor in Young Living by purchasing the Basic Starter Kit for $40 or the Starter Kit for $75. The Basic Kit includes a bottle of Stress Away, 2 samples (2 oz) of Ningxia Red, and a few samples of oils. The Starter Kit adds a diffuser to the mix. We don't suggest either scenario, because the set of oils you receive (10 in the Everyday Kit, in addition to the Stress Away that also comes in the other kits) in the Premium Starter Kit are the best part of Young Living. You have to use them to be able to share them. I do mention this, though, because you can get in to Young Living cheaper than the $150. This would enable someone to start teaching classes, and getting enrollments, and earning Fast Start bonuses for a minimal investment- as low as $40. The only drawback I can conceive is that it may be difficult to share about the oils if you don't have any to use. Just my thoughts…

[214] *The Four Year Career,* Kindle Version, location 133.

[215] For instance, if you are going to earn $4,000 / month as a distributor, for instance ($48,000 / year) you would need a $1,000,000 investment earning 5% a year to meet that income. If you had $1,000,000 sitting around, you probably wouldn't need a home-based business or the extra income.

☐ _____

☐ _____

☐ _____

Want to know more?

☐ Read:

☐ *The Four Year Career: How to Make Your Dreams Fun and Financial Freedom Come True... or Not*, by Richard Bliss Brooke

☐ "Oils that Heal vs Oils that Don't," Chapter 13 in *Healing Oils of the Bible*, David Stewart.

☐ Listen:

☐ To the relevant chapter of the audiobook

☐ Search:

☐ Direct Selling Association (DSA)- DSA.org - a "professional group that represents and sets standards for the Network Marketing Industry."[216]

---

[216] *The Four Year Career*, Kindle location 589, suggests this as a site to research.

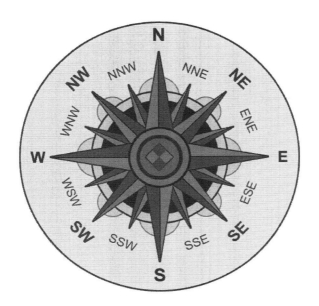

04: Try something new / Les's story

I remember when we first heard about Young Living Essential oils. We were living paycheck to paycheck- always looking for ways to make ends meet, keep food on the table, and save enough to get away for a weekend every now and then. Small changes in our budget made big deals in our daily life.

When our thirteen year old was two we learned as young parents what it was like to have a child with asthma. We have had a couple of week-long visits to the hospital when her asthma got out of control.

Les Wright has been married to Kelli for 17 years. They have 2 daughters, and have been members of Young Living since September 2012.

Along the way we also learned that she was allergic to several things that showed up as eczema. This not only caused us to have a constant battle with both of these issues, but also kept us on our toes fighting these ailments every day. Over the years, doctors prescribed several kinds of medications to mask or lessen the symptoms for both of these issues. Each time something new was prescribed, it came with a warning.These prescriptions, even when used as directed, were either bad for her internally or externally, or they wound up being ineffective. We found ourselves using these medications, out of desperation. We felt like it was the only option.

In addition to the harm we knew that this could cause daughter's health, the trips to the doctor, the medications, and the chaos was a huge strain on our already tight finances. When you are faced with relief for your child or a vacation or new clothes, relief for your child ALWAYS always comes first.

And what I described above was our reality for almost 10 years! We had accepted this as our way of life. Then an amazing thing happened....We were battling an extremely bad case of eczema that had become infected in some areas. When the doctor told my wife that the medications he recommended were harmful if we continued to use them, she began asking around for advice and prayer.

Some of our friends had been using products from Young Living with amazing success. They suggested Lavender and Melrose Oils along with Lavender Lotion and Rose Ointment. Well, the skeptic in me really doubted, but my wife did a great job of being persistent and getting them ordered. It was done and we had an order placed for a natural remedy. We ordered some oil!

I remember the first night the products arrived. My daughter was lying on the couch as my wife carefully applied the oils. Our friends were great about helping us understand how to use them, but I had huge doubts. Honestly, I believed we were wasting time and money. We had been walking this road of illness for solong, we really didn't expect much in the way of results. Then my daughter's eczema infection actually looked a little worse the next day!

Instead of quitting my wife jumped into research mode. She found that this was actually a good thing and was the start of the healing process. She was right. Within a week, the areas were much better and our daughter even knew how to apply the products to make sure eczema was a thing of the past.

As the weeks and months passed, we learned about a couple other oils that helped control the asthma. Now, our whole family is into different types of Young Living oils. We use them for a huge variety of things from fever to headaches to toothpaste to a great energy booster. The products are very versatile and we have seen them work for us. They have the additional benefit of being pure. To me, pure means eliminating so many of the side effects we worried about for so many years.

And not to mention the COSTS of these medications. After one year of using the Young Living products for my daughter, we saw a savings of a little more than $700 in medical costs. In our house that was a much needed savings.

I am confident that God used our friends to introduce us to these products at the perfect time. We were in a place where we needed help and were open to trying something we may not have in the past. I am thankful that they were willing to share their story with us and help us.

If I could encourage anyone through our journey with oils I would say jump in and learn more. Looking back, I would love to say I was the one that joined in with my wife and learned about the products.

You're probably intrigued by now so, my advice is to study what doctors are saying. Try one or two for yourself. Start small and form your own opinion. Be creative in trying new things.

— Les Wright, Kelli's husband

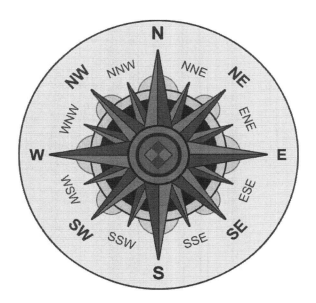

05: Getting traction

I hope you're making time to do some of the action steps I've suggested along this journey- and that you've been reading and listening and searching out some of the information I've pointed you towards... My hope is that this book doesn't merely impart information to you, but that it leads to some sort of, dare I say it, change... a *transformation*, of sorts.

Here's the journey I've taken you on so far:

> *The main idea:* There are practical ways to support your wife. It's not just about learning information, though, it's about implementing what you are learning, and putting some things into practice.

- We've discussed the leadership and culture of Young Living. I've told you about my personal interaction with the founder and some of the stories I've heard.

- We've looked at a brief history of essential oils, including an extensive look at when and where the oils are used throughout Scripture.

- We've talked about what these essential oils are- and evaluated what makes Young Living a better grade than another.

- We've looked at multilevel marketing. I've detailed for you why I believe network marketing provides a fantastic business opportunity for you.

If you're still reading, I'm assuming you're still interested. So, **in this part of the book I'm going to provide you with a few practical ways-** *things you can actually do-* **to begin supporting your wife in this new venture.** Some of these things will be easy, others will take a bit of work. Don't let any single thing here overwhelm you- think incremental steps, because *a series of little steps equates to major change.* Besides, I think with a little bit of intentionality, you'll be able to thread each of them into your regular routine.

"Tell them, that. . ."

When we returned from Hawaii, we invited two dear friends, Kent and Stacy (people in our upline) on a double date to discuss the trip: what we learned, what we saw. And, of course, everyone always wants to know what Gary is like in real life! My wife scheduled the dinner date three or four days after we returned, so I already had an outline sketched out for this book. And I knew that a significant part of the book would be the testimonials from other guys whom I was planning to include.

I knew Kent was one of the guys I wanted in the book. He and Stacy have been doing the business for almost a year and have been successful in their efforts. In fact, she had a house cleaning business she started years ago. The oil business began taking so much time and generating more income so she decided it was time to set the other business aside. Kent is a State Trooper who's almost vested, meaning he probably won't quit until he caps that out, regardless of the success Stacy has with Young Living. It just wouldn't make sense, because he can draw a retirement check for the rest of his life after he hits a certain mark. I tell you that to show you that **there's no "right way" or "wrong way" to plan your future. It's your future. Not mine. Not someone else's.** You get to plan it in the way that works best for your family.

Somewhere during dinner, I told Kent about the book, and asked if he would be willing to share his story about how he got involved with the oils; and pass on any info he thought would be helpful for other guys.

That led us to a conversation about a few things. Stacy was doing well- and was now surpassing his salary. And mine. She was the highest paid person sitting at the table.

"One of the guys I met in Hawaii told me that his dad asked him how he felt about his wife making a bigger check than he was…" I offered.

Kent laughed and wanted to know what the guy said.

"The guy told his dad that they used to be a one income family. He knew what his check was and that they had been able to pay all of the bills with it and had been doing OK. Not fantastic, but everything always got

> That's how you roll when the "bigger check" issue comes up. You simply smile and say, "Thanks."

paid… He told his dad it would be crazy to be upset that she had experienced significant success and was now making *four times* what he was making each month. Why would he be mad at that? It left his dad speechless…"

Kent laughed again and then offered- "I would just say… if somebody asked me what I do when Stacy makes more than I do… I just take the check to the bank and cash it. That's how we handle that! We say thank you and we accept it."

In other words, for Kent- and all the guys I've talked with, for that matter- it's not a big deal.

Kent had some other advice. He started off with, "You tell all of the guys when you write this book that…"

I interrupted him.

"Hey, wait. I want *you* to tell them. Will you write it up for me?" I said. "Seriously. Tell them anything…"

So, you'll hear from Kent in the next testimonial. By the way, the check came and Kent decided the person who made the most money should pay. We grinned and passed the check to Stacy.

She beamed with a wide smile that lights up her entire face, grabbed the check with the good kind of pride, and told us, "I've got it boys."

Neither one of us were too prideful to let her get it, either. That's how you roll when the "bigger check" issue comes up. You simply smile and say, "Thanks."

That said, here's my top 7 ways you can get traction and start helping your wife *right now*, even today:

- #1- Become your wife's best customer

- #2- Read two books about essential oils

- #3- Download a podcast

- #4- Find someone to tell you a few things that have worked for them- about the oils or the business, either one

- #5- Go and see something (Young Living sponsored event)

- #6- Pick one way to help your wife

- #7- Understand the compensation plan

Let's move through each of these over the next few pages.

#1- Become your wife's best customer

No, I don't mean that you should go buy a bunch of stuff from her. She already spends some of your family's hard-earned money each month or you wouldn't be this deep into the book, I'm guessing. She might have even bought the book for you, proving my point that she's already reaching out for support."

Here's what I suggest you do: find *a few* oils that will work for you- and start using them.

If you're like I was before going to Hawaii, you haven't been using *anything* (except likely Valor that *she* is putting on your big toe or spine so she can sleep at night without the roar of a snore), so this will all be new to you. If you already have a few "go to" oils, you're ahead of the curve. Either way, I've provided you with a list of a few ways to get started. If you have a few tricks up your sleeve, send them to me and I'll post them online or put them in the next edit of this book.

Some of my go to uses for oils and YL products

What I use	Diffuse when	Apply topically	Notes
Endoflex		After working out	Cristy mixed this with some lotion that I can use to massage my muscles after working out or a long run- as a result, I rarely have soreness.
Lavender		Sunburns and bites	
Peppermint	I want a cheery atmosphere in the office	Stings	
Lemon			I also drop this in water to drink- or in Ningxia Red.
Purification		Insect Repellant	
Panaway		Sore or stiff muscles	
Vetiver	Lower stress / anxiety, chill things out…	Lower stress / anxiety	I diffuse this when one of my rowdy boys is with me; I also carry it in my pocket (the 5ml bottle) when he is with me, giving him a few whiffs throughout the day.
Peace and calming	Same as Vetiver	Sleep	Diffuse when the little, rowdy boys are around.
Ningxia Red			Drink twice a day, morning and evening, 2 oz.
Power Meal	n/a	n/a	I began using this as a meal replacement, as part of my weight reduction plan. It tastes, well, like a protein shake. However, it's actually good with about 2 oz of Ningxia Red mixed in!
Thieves	Diffuse at the office, great aroma and purifies the air		We use this as our commercial grade cleaner at The Village- it kills shower scum, we get 100 Health ratings for cleanliness in the kitchen, etc.

Anyway, those are some of my uses. You'll figure out your own. There are guys I'm on a FaceBook group with that constantly mix oils with Ningxia Red, trying various concoctions for anything and everything you can think of. They're ahead of me in the game- and may stay there, as far as mixing "oil drinks" is concerned. My point is this: do what works for you. Experiment and have fun. You've already got the oils, anyway, and I'm sure she'll be glad for you to touch them.

Plus, you will feel "more a part" of what your wife is doing- and she'll certainly feel like you're "more a part" of things once you thread YL products throughout your daily routine.

#2- Go read two books

There's a lot of great stuff that's been written. In the intro chapter I suggested you go on a media fast for a short period of time, simply so you could "de-clutter" your mind and absorb things that are more important for a brief season. Now is the time to pick something up. Go grab something and read it. You'll look smarter, you'll learn a bit, and you'll get bonus points around the house. Carrying that book around will be like having a little halo in your hip pocket.

Here are a few suggestions:

- For now, read the introductory chapters to the *Essential Oils Pocket Reference*. You can access the remaining 90% of the book when you "need to know" something specific.

- If you want to improve your overall health and fitness, pick up Scott's book *TransformWise.*

- If you like studying your Bible, grab *Healing Oils of the Bible*- or something like that.

There are books out there on pet care, babies, and just about everything else re: essential oils.

Francis Bacon said, "Reading makes a man go wide; writing makes a man go deep."

Later, there may be a time to go deep- for yourself or for others. You may want to jot down ways you can use the oils while hunting, as part of your exercise regimen, or even in grilling out (yes, you can use them for all of that). For now, though, you probably need to "go wide" to get exposed to the various things the oils can do.

#3- Download a podcast

You can't learn everything, so my suggestion is to learn *some* things. I know you're busy- probably too busy to take on another thing. My advice is that you "stack" you're learning with something else you're already doing.

> You don't have to take notes, and you won't be tested. You'll be surprised at how much you'll retain.

- If you drive to work, stack your learning with your commute.

- If you run for exercise, stack it.

- If you fish… well… I won't go that far…

Here's the deal: you can learn a lot in a short amount of time if you download something that's taught by someone who's smart. So go grab a few audio files, put them on your phone or mp3 player and start learning. You don't have to take notes, and you won't be tested. You'll be surprised at how much you'll retain.

Cristy knows her way around the computer, but she admits to being technologically challenged in some ways. As we were prepping for our trip to Hawaii she asked if I would download a few podcasts about essential oils to her iPad. I searched online and, with the traction that essential oils have gotten lately, was honestly surprised there weren't *more* out there than there were. I was successful, though, and found enough to occupy her time.

Of course, I chose some I thought she might like- and I selected a few I thought I might like for her to have:

- "Essential oils for family health" for her.

- "Spring cleansing" for her.

- "Health children" for her.

- "The libido and essential oils" *for me.*

Yep, that's where I learned that there truly was an oil for everything. Yes, even that. (My wife insists I add that she learned quite a bit about how adrenal function plays into libido. But you'll have to listen to it to learn more.)

#4- Find someone to tell you a few things

A few pages back, I talked about the laborers in the field- that there were amazing people already working the Young Living plot of land and that you had been invited to their party. Rather than complaining like the guys did in Jesus' version of the parable, all of the distributors I've met at Young Living have been more than happy to share their experience with me and let me stand on their shoulders and take a peek around.

About a week ago, I called Les. You just met him a few pages ago. His wife is one of the new-breed rockstars that started The Lemon Droppers. We're on their team.

"I need some help…" I told him on the phone.

"Sure. Anything. What's up?"

I went on to explain that Cristy had started getting checks that were somewhat significant in size, and that I was starting to budget and plan. "We're setting a specific bit of money aside for Cristy to put back into her business each month… and we're putting a specific percentage aside for taxes…"

"You're on the right track," he told me.

I explained, "I know you guys learned this through experience. You're about 18 months ahead of us… I'd simply like to hear what you've learned and save myself the time trying to learn it. I'll borrow your research and just do whatever you found out we're supposed to do with taxes and everything…"

> … all of the distributors I've met at Young Living have been more than happy to share their experience with me and let me stand on their shoulders and take a peek around.

And there it was. He was glad to help; I was glad to take the help. Les even offered to let me sit down with him and his accountant in the next few weeks after that conversation. He was happy to help.

Here's my point. **There are guys who've figured out everything you're trying to learn right now. You don't have to go search for answers they've already found.** Yes, it's good to find your own way in life and determine what your own worldview is and to discover certain things on your own that can only be learned by experience.

Understanding taxes and getting basic information about how the oils work and what the business model is *are not* some of those things that you need to necessarily figure out on your own. Why reinvent the wheel? Learn from the other guys who've already done it. Get inside someone else's head and peak around.

Here's a non-oil related example: I have an orange Nikon CoolPix camera that I carry around when we travel. I bought it because my brother-in-law, Frank, studies every possible scenario before he buys a gadget. When it was time for me to buy one, I just asked him what he would buy. Then I trusted his research and bought what he told me he would buy himself. End of story. Was that irresponsible? Absolutely not. He knows more about cameras and gadgets than I ever will, so his decision is well-informed. Plus, I spent the afternoon watching a football game with my dad instead of surfing the Internet.

I'll tell you where I've learned a lot about oils: FaceBook. That's right. One of the guys in our upline, Verick, started a guys group. He added me. I've added some others. I talk with those guys 3-5 times a day. I've learned a great deal about the oils from them- and probably more about life.

> Understanding taxes and getting basic information about how the oils work and what the business model is *are not* some of those things that you need to necessarily figure out on your own.

By way of example here are two things we learned simply by talking to others:

We learned about the Leadership Development Credit program. Under this program, Young Living allowed distributors who hit a certain rank to obtain a few kits on consignment. If you've enrolled people within 30 days, you would give them the kit and Young Living would drop ship a new one to you- instead of to the new distributor. Then your 30 day clock would re-start.

Now, you know as well as I do, that people are more likely to enroll when they see that kit in front of them and can pay and take it with them. They don't "go home and think about it" as often. And then they don't have to wait for it to come in the mail before they can start using the products. They leave excited, with the merchandise, and they're ready to jam.

We also learned about virtual classes. Not webinars, but virtual classes. I mentioned this earlier, too. A virtual class is simply a short film that you shoot of yourself teaching what you would teach in person. People can log on to watch your movie, or they can hold a meeting where multiple people watch it together.

There are many incredible ideas out there and many practical things you need to know. Don't try to figure them out by yourself. No sense in trying to discover fire. That's already been done. Just sit down and talk with a few guys- or message back and forth- and you're good to go.

#5- Go and see something

One of the best things you can do, to see if Young Living is right for you or not, is to attend an actual event. Better yet, while you're there, go talk to Gary (tell him I sent you) and ask him any question in the world about anything. He'll smile, he'll probably hug you, and then he'll talk to you as long as you want to stand there and talk. I'm being serious.

There's nothing like going first hand to see something. Disney is different than watching Mickey Mouse in your house. A live football game is better than even watching things play out on a big screen television. Concerts are better then iPod playlists, and seeing Young Living in person is better than hearing about it from afar.

Don't misunderstand. You can learn a lot online, by reading a book, or by listening to a recording. But there is something special about interacting with the real people. That's where you learn the culture and values in a tangible way. I thought Young Living was going to be a lot of hype, and assumed they "over did" things just like most other successful companies. You know the routine, you go into a large banquet hall and people are all cheering and going all rah-rah about some product.

The Ningxia event, the place where I wore the t-shirt, confirmed my suspicion: it was a lot of hype. At the same time, the event also confirmed something else: it was a lot of substance, too. I discovered that the two- hype/cheer/rah-rah and substance aren't mutually exclusive. But for me, it took seeing it in person to understand that. In addition, you meet incredible people at the events- folks that you would never meet otherwise. And you find out that you have a lot in common with them, and that you're on a similar journey.

Spencer and Cristina are two such people. They live in San Diego where Spencer is a photojournalist for NBC. His trade is so bred into him that he actually clicks his phone to "video" mode when boarding a

> ... values and culture and honor aren't always "taught" with words- they're "caught" through experience.

plane or going to a public place- just so that he's ready to capture anything exciting that happens spontaneously. He wore Go Pro cameras when zip lining in Hawaii. He never misses anything.

Cristina, like Cristy, is a doula and assists with natural childbirth. They've been involved with Young Living about the same amount of time as we have. In fact, Cristina hit Gold two days before Cristy did- before Cristy did the first time, anyway (I'll give you the back story on that in the next chapter).

Anyway, a bunch of us went zip lining in Hawaii. Cristina was chatting with our guide, a female about 20 years old. She found out the guide had sore shoulders and a few other ailments that had been bothering her for a few weeks. So guess what? Cristina pulled out her oils and healed the girl- right there! It was awesome.

What's the point? Getting around people who *lead* an organization *and* people who are *involved* in the organization teaches you a great deal. Honestly, it teaches you more than words can communicate, because values and culture and honor aren't always "taught" with words- they're "caught" through experience.

#6- Pick something to do

My first nose dive into essential oils was a teaching video I edited for Cristy. She's an amazing teacher. The only problem is that she can't be out of the house every night of the week. As well, she has people that live outside of Alabama that can't make it to her classes when she offers them.

Enter the video class idea.

Now, my wife has a certain way of wanting things done, *even when I'm doing things for her.* If you're a wife reading this book you might know what I mean when I say that. And it's likely that you, husbands, are laughing because you, *too*, know *exactly* what I mean.

My concrete, man-mind thinking is this: you can tell me what you want done or you can do it. But you can't do both. If you're going to ask me to do it, step out of the way and let me do it, so I can get back to what I was doing. Even if I was just chilling out on the couch doing nothing more when you recruited me for your task. I know, it may sound barbaric. But I'm just being real, here.

So she wants to make a video. Or, better yet, she wants to record herself talking on video via our desktop computer in the dimly lit guest bedroom down stairs, and then she wants me to craft it into something Oscar-worthy. (My wife is editing this book, and wants you all to know that this is not entirely how it went down. But she's going to leave my version of the story in here, since it's my book.)

If you've ever edited something, you know it's a pain in the *rumpus maximus*. It takes about one hour of work for every 1-2 minutes of editing you're doing- no matter how simple the project appears to be. That means a 30-minute video should take you about 15-30 hours. Cristy thought it would take about an hour. Like I could wave a wand in the back room, walk out, and boom!

I'll be honest with you: I fussed, screamed, nagged and about pulled my hair out trying to get that thing done. That's just being real.

Yet, at the end of the day I should have bypassed the murmuring because this was the end result:

- The video was completed. It took me about 15 hours total time to do it (so I finished it on the fast side of the projection).

- That training film saved her *more* than the 15 hours in travel time, teaching time, and planning time. This meant more time together for other things.

- The movie generated in excess of 1/3 of our total enrollments to this date, meaning it helped kick-start our business into high gear.

- We continue to use it *even now*. Sure, we've learned more about the oils since that first film was created (I knew basically *nothing* about them when I edited it for her), but we haven't had time to make a better replacement. That one still works. We'll make another when we have a chance to do it. Until then, it continues working on our behalf and helps others learn the basics of essential oils and Young Living.

Now, you may not be an editing wizard or an A/V techie, but I guarantee you that you're awesome at something. Pick one thing that you're good at; something that would help your wife's business, and do it.

Answer the FaceBook questions that people ask over and over and over again. You'll learn more about what the oils do in the process.

> You got the idea- and you've probably already come up with something *better* than what I've suggested. Just find your thing and do it.

Or research questions people have for her about how to treat certain health issues with the oils. The time spent digging through the *Essential Oils Pocket Reference* will help her, encourage her team and free her to spend more time with you and the kids.

Or deliver books and oils to people, if that's what she needs you to do. Get the kids out of the house so she has some uninterrupted time to actually run the business, take the kids to get ice cream, and make the oil deliveries on the way.

Or take the oils to work and share them with people who need them.[217] Troubleshoot their aches and pains and help them find something that works for them. You got the idea- and you've probably already come up with something *better* than what I've suggested. Just find your thing and do it.

#7- Understand the compensation plan

By the end of the first morning in Hawaii, I had seen that things would probably hum along a lot smoother and quicker if I found out *how* I could help Cristy. A few pages ago, I introduced you to James, the pastor. Since he is a man I respect, I asked him how long they had been involved with the "business side" of YL, and how he came to help Stacy. Like us- and like most couples involved in Young Living- his wife originally "did things on her own" and later welcomed his help when he was ready to give it.

He laughed when I asked the question. Then- "Well, for the first 10 months or so, I didn't do *anything* with Young Living at all."

---

[217] Because I'm "the boss" in my office, I consider it kosher for anything Young Living to be used at my workplace.

His story already sounded familiar, I told him. He went on to say that at some point someone encouraged them that the best way to build their business was to simply "sign people up" with a minimal order and then let things happen naturally. In other words, there was no strategy involved. So, Stacy was holding meetings, teaching people about the oils (she's an incredible communicator, by the way), and signing a few people up. It kept her pretty busy, but not very profitable.

"At the end of those ten months," James continued, "Stacy was making about $50 a month."

By now, my wife and Stacy, who had been discussing kids and catching up, were paying attention. They decided to chime in.

"He told me I should look at *quitting*," Stacy said.

James concurred. "It was taking *soooo* much time," he elaborated. "She was exhausted. I was tired. And I actually gave her a few suggestions for more books she should write instead of spending her time with the oils."

It seemed, from hearing them, that they were going to still use the products, they were just going to move away from the business side. After all, with no plan, and with no direction, trying to run a business *can* be exhausting.

"That's when Stacy reminded me of something," James continued. "She reminded me that I once told her a few months before then that we needed to study the compensation plan, to really study and learn how you make money from the business side of things. Up to that point, I had not yet done that."

He agreed that he would study the compensation plan throughout the month of October. If he found a way to make it work profitably, they would continue with the business in November. If he didn't, they would quit.

"I studied it, we implemented what we learned, and we've never looked back," they said. He explained that the check amounts went up immediately and continued to climb. Today, they are compensated more than they ever imagined. Because of this income, they have more options for ministry *and* writing *and* an ease in life that suits them well.

James' advice is good: *study the compensation plan and learn how it is that you get paid.*

I know. It seems so obvious. **In every line of work, for every single employer you've ever had (or every employee you've ever had, if you're the boss), the question is always the same:** *How and when do I get paid?* It's surprising how many people overlook the financial incentives when they evaluate MLMs, though. Somehow, a lot of people (especially husbands like me, who were sitting "outside" looking in) never apply that same logic to an independent distributorship with Young Living.

Once you understand the compensation plan, you'll get an idea how many classes you need to teach in order to grow your team. You'll also see how long it may take your wife to earn a certain size paycheck. And it will help you plan, now, as you prepare to move forward into a more financially-free future.

> In every line of work, for every single employer you've ever had (or every employee you've ever had, if you're the boss), the question is always the same: *How and when do I get paid?*

So how do you get paid? I don't have the space to show you in this chapter. So, I've written a detailed overview of the compensation plan as a resource guide that supplements this book. You can find it on the website.

The next step

That's it. Those are my seven ways to get traction and start walking this thing out with your wife.

I know, you may feel like you have a long way to go. **Just remember, incremental change, over time, is exponential.** Don't feel like you have to do all seven today- just start doing something. Then do a little more after that, then a bit more after that.

Over time, you'll peek in the rearview mirror and marvel at how far you've traveled. And, you'll feel like a team because you'll be moving with her in something she loves doing. That will make it worth every step of the journey.

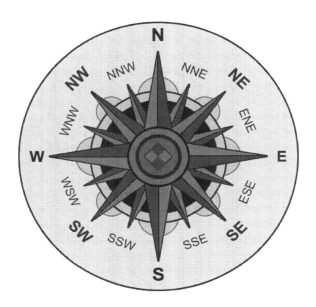

05: Direction: know how it works

Action steps

> **The main idea:** There are practical ways to support your wife. It's not just about learning information, though, it's about implementing what you are learning, and putting some things into practice.

☐ Most people give up before they succeed. In other words, the "success" (however you define it in your own terms) may be just around the corner. If you write down what you're willing to do, or your goals, you won't grow weary.

☐ Define where you want to be.

☐ Go through the list of seven things you can do to help your wife. Write what you'll do for each of these:

   ☐ Become your wife's best customer

- [ ] Read two books
- [ ] Download a podcast
- [ ] Find someone to tell you a few things that have worked for them- regarding the business or the oils
- [ ] Go and see something
- [ ] Pick one way to help your wife- something you will do
- [ ] Learn the compensation plan

Want to know more?

- [ ] Read:
  - [ ] "Young Living Essential Oils Compensation Plan: Enjoying Abundance" (this is a trifold, four-color brochure, produced by Young Living, item number 4720).
  - [ ] "Young Living Terms and Definitions for the Compensation Plan" (PDF document, 9 pages in length).
- [ ] Listen:
  - [ ] Go online to www.OurSimpleTraining.com/Monday-Night-Calls and listen to conference call from March 10, 2014, on compensation.
  - [ ] Young Living Education podcast.[218]
  - [ ] To the relevant chapter of the audiobook
- [ ] Search:
  - [ ] Go to your wife's virtual office. Yes, this will require getting her to show you how to login using her password. Trust me, if you have this book and have made it this far she

---

[218] https://itunes.apple.com/us/podcast/young-living-education/id303198270?mt=2 - this is the podcast I referenced in the chapter that has the episode about the libido.

will be *thrilled* to give it to you and show you around. There you should familiarize with each of the following:

☐ PowerPoint

☐ James McDonald and his wife, Stacy, created the following videos to explain the compensation plan. They are worth your time to watch & review- and have been placed here with their permission.[219]

☐ "Starting a Young Living Business," 39:22 minutes, located at https://vimeo.com/68374318

☐ "The Rising Star Bonus!" 6:30 minutes, at https://vimeo.com/71178056

☐ "The Accidental Paycheck," 6:33 minutes, at https://vimeo.com/74031607

---

[219] Their website is www.CommonScentsMom.com

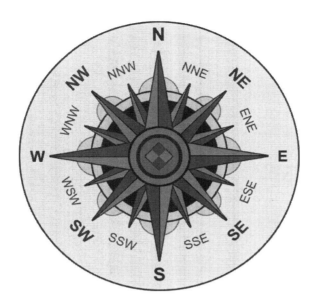

05: It almost seems unfair... / Josh's story

Growing up, everything I had heard about recovering from sickness and injury was directly influenced by my family. And most of them worked in the hospital as medical professionals. So, to say conventional medicine was ingrained in us pretty heavily would be a pretty accurate statement.

Fast forward to about 12-13 years ago, to when I met my wife, Fredia. At the time she was studying to be a nurse and was finishing up all of her college work. After we starting

Josh Nelms has been married to Fredia for 10 years. They have three young children and have been involved with Young Living since November 2013.

dating, I quickly discovered that she wasn't your typical nurse. She always had a desire to study and understand more natural and organic ways of handling diet, medical treatment, childbirth, etc. I remember on many occasions, when I wasn't feeling well, she would want to treat my ailments with remedies I'd have to buy at the local heath food store or vitamin shop. She was clearly ahead of the curve on this sort of thing. Much more than anyone else that I had known.

During the Fall of 2013, Fredia was introduced to Young Living essential oils. This was not my wife's first encounter with oils, but my wife was very excited to find a company that manufactured quality oils with the attention to detail that Young Living provided. After trying some of the oils, she was hooked, and ordered her Premium Kit. Being the somewhat reluctant person that I am, I proceeded with caution into the world of "snake oils" as my brother-in-law and I like to refer to them.

We started out by using Peace and Calming on our children to help with sleeping and staying grounded. Our daughter gets Vetiver and Orange on a daily basis to help her focus and stay emotionally grounded. We all use different oils for daily aches and pains as well. AND my children love taking their NingXia every morning.

Fredia began to use Valor on me regularly, so I would stop snoring and both of us could sleep better. When anyone in the family starting showing signs of flu, she would make up Thieves capsules for us, to either shorten the time affected, or usually prevent sickness. Now, when I feel like something is not right, I'll tell her what is going on, and she'll give me something to take or apply.

After a Zyto scan to point out more specific issues going on with my body, I started using Present Time to help with focus and balance during the day. I've also starting drinking Ningxia Red to help with focus and energy levels, and a Nitro boost when I know I'm going to have a long day. I've been shocked by how much better I feel. Have I mentioned that even my immediate family have started using the oils and are seeing amazing results?

Since I'm slow to learn which oils help certain ailments, it's nice to be able to get my wife's suggestions on certain oils. If she doesn't know the answer, the amazing community of Young Living oil users is always quick to provide some helpful suggestions as well. It's amazing to me how so many different oils can be used for different treatments. And when you start combining the oils, it seems like there is an almost endless possibility of ways to use these oils.

Being a Young Living distributor has been a huge blessing to my wife and me. We love helping others find alternative ways of treatment and healthy living. It's encouraging to see her light up when she tells me about how someone is going to start using to oils and it's helping them, or how they're able (by their choice) to stop taking some medication because of it. It makes it even better that we are able to earn an income from this. It almost seems unfair to be getting paid to help others out, but that is part of the beauty of Young Living.

Our family loves the oils, and believes in the healing power of them. We hope to be able to share this with all of our friends and family.

– Josh Nelms, Fredia's husband

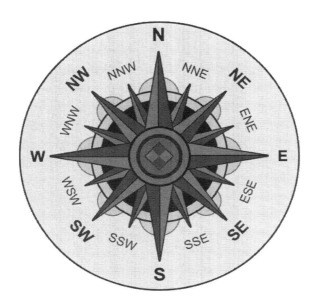

06: Reverse engineer your life

Have you ever noticed that a lot of things in life seem to happen by chance or accident? Or certainly by God's blessing. You don't plan, you don't prepare. It just happens: Some bit of goodness just comes your way.

I'm grateful for good surprises, like free tickets to the carnival. We received those a few weeks ago. Somebody called, they happened to be working at the large fair that came through town, and the owner allowed them to toss tickets our way. We arrived, the owner and his wife came and met us- and all nine kids- and the owner's wife told the kids to come see her for free cotton candy after they had fun riding all the rides they could handle.

> **The main idea:** Your destination is determined by the direction you are headed. Decide where you want to go, plan your course, and start stepping in that direction.

Sitting atop the ferris wheel, I marveled at it all. People were paying $20.00 for wrist bands that provided an unlimited pass to all of the attractions. We had 10 of them- because the baby clearly wasn't going to ride in anything except his hiking backpack. People were plopping down $7.00 for cotton candy. Each of the eight participating kids had been offered their own free of charge. We weren't expecting anything and had been given a $256.00 night of fun. No charge. I'm grateful for surprises like that one. And I take them with deep gratitude when they come.

While these blessings seem to find their way to us time and time again, with nine kids, Cristy and I still do a great deal of planning, preparing, saving and working towards goals. We live with a budget, we schedule our weeks, and we evaluate extracurricular activities before we commit to them, we save for vacations and vehicles. Planning is not a bad thing. In fact, I'm learning that good preparation often frees us up to receive even more blessings!

Here's what I've learned:

- Most things work smoother when there's an actual plan.

- The plan can always change. In other words, you're not held hostage by your own plan.[220]

- Your destination, where you end up, is most often determined by what you were already doing- not by the random things that happen along the path.

That last one is important- that **the trajectory of your life, the decisions you make and things you do every single day, have far more to do with how things go for you than random chance and luck.**

Your destination is determined by your direction

I told you earlier in the book that I jumped full throttle into an exercise and weight loss regiment. Actually, it was more of an "eating right" regiment. I was already exercising. I did most of the P90X regimen and actually *gained* weight. Whereas you see the before and after shots of everyone on television and marvel at how much slimmer they become, I went in the opposite direction. I actually packed on the pounds.

---

[220] Ironically, this is why a lot of people absolutely refuse to create a budget. I tell them, "It's your plan for how you want to spend your money. You decide where your money goes. You can change it if you want, because you created it and the plan is there to serve you and your needs."

I was overweight because, no matter how much I wanted to be fit, two caramel mochas or vanilla lattes a day, along with assorted candies and pastries throughout the day, seconds after every meal, followed by a late night snack don't lead to "lean and fit." That road leads to festively plump, right where I found myself.

Here's one of the most brilliant statements I've ever heard about this topic: "Your direction- not your intention- determines your destination."[221] In other words, **you end up where you are headed, regardless of whether or not you wanted to end up there.** You may need to read that sentence again. It sounds odd, because it's so overly obvious.

> The truth is simply this: My direction is what determines my destination.

Think about it like this: If I want to travel from Alabama to Tennessee, I must drive north. If I drive south, regardless of how much I want to go to Tennessee, I will never arrive there. The only thing that will help is *if I change my direction.*

- My intentions will not help.

- More praying will not help.

- Having more faith will not help.

- My IQ will not help.

- My background will not help (whether it be religious upbringing, practical experience, or even economic status).

- Seeing the "bright side" and having a positive outlook won't help.

- Even having friends and family encourage me to "keep at it" won't do anything to get me there.

Why will I end up in Tennessee if I go north? **Because that's where that road heads.** Why will I not end up in Tennessee if I drive south? Because that road ends up somewhere else.

The truth is simply this: **My direction is what determines my destination.** The road you are on determines where you go for no other reasons than:

---

[221] See Andy Stanley's book *The Principle of the Path,*

- You are on that road, *and*

- That's where that road goes.

This concept is easy to grasp when you consider it from the perspective of driving somewhere. However, it's often difficult to see that the same concept that applies to moving forward down the highway also applies to moving forward through life. If you find yourself on the wrong road while driving (let's say it's still the same road from Alabama to Tennessee, but you accidentally drove south towards Florida instead), you have a few options: You can:

- Change directions and make it to your destination (i.e., put it in reverse, do a U-turn in the middle of the road, catch the next exit and turn around). *Or,*

- Continue in the same direction and miss your destination.

Changing directions on the Interstate is easy. In life, the transition might not be so simple: "Worst case [in driving], you've wasted a few minutes or hours. But when you get lost in life, you can't backtrack. When you get lost in life, you don't waste minutes or hours. You can waste an entire season of your life. Choosing the wrong path in life will cost you precious years..."[222] Sure, you can learn from experience ("I guess I'll just have to learn it the hard way," some people say), but experience eats up the most valuable asset you have- *time*. It makes more sense to just "plan ahead" and map the course.

Reverse engineer your life

Since our destination (where we end up) is determined by the direction we head), **doesn't it make sense that we could decide where we want to end up and then build a map of how to get there?** Couldn't we "start at the end" and plot all the steps necessary in order to make it where we want to be?

The answer is, simply, "Yes."

We do this when we go places where we have never been. You type the address into Google maps (or into an "map app" on your smartphone), you research the Internet to find restaurants and hotels in the area, and you begin plotting your course. You don't just head in *any* direction- you head in the direction that takes

---

[222] *The Principle of the Path*, page 33.

you where you want to go. We do this when doing something as simple as moving to a new house. You look ahead and decide which room in the new house you want to function as the bedroom, which one would be the den, etc. Then, you pack your belongings in labelled boxes and route them to the proper destination. You did this if you've been to college and plotted a future career. You might have known that you needed certain classes, a specific internship, or some sort of resume builder in order to land the job you wanted.

In all of the examples above, **you didn't simply pray harder or desire the change, you actually made plans and worked the plans towards the intended destination**. You understand, even if you didn't have the words to articulate it, your destination is determined by your direction. And, yes, you probably

> Since our destination (where we end up) is determined by the direction we head), doesn't it make sense that we could decide where we want to end up and then build a map of how to get there?

prayed & believed & had faith & looked on the bright side of things & had people cheering you on, too.

Here's the oddity, though- *We rarely do this with life-as-a-whole even though the same principle is true*:

- If you are going to marry one kind of spouse, that eliminates a bunch of others. In other words, if you want a woman (or man) who has the same values as you, who desires to not fall into the same vices that have ensnared you before, then those facts alone eliminate masses of people.

- If you want your children to grow up in a certain way- and be able to manage their home by keeping their house clean, keeping a chore schedule, and responding to others with honor and respect- you should train them in that way now.

- If you want to spend your days working in a job that fulfills your calling rather than just provides you with a paycheck, you will likely need to be intentional about it. You will need to evaluate what jobs are available, determine what certifications or training you need, and then act accordingly. Tim Ferriss wrote a book about this, *The 4-Hour Work Week*. In that book he argues that you shouldn't wait for retirement to enjoy life. Rather, you should intentionally look at opportunities to move from the daily grind into daily fulfillment now. If that is something you desire, you will have to be intentional.[223]

Here's the reality: **If you do not plan life, it will still happen.** And rather than heading in a direction that you intend, you will likely end up in some other direction. As well, you'll likely find yourself in some random destination, then sit scratching your head and wondering how you ever got *there* (I've done this plenty of times while driving *and in life*). In life, just as in driving, it's often difficult to determine just where it was that you went off-course and started getting lost. Most often, it just occurs that you're somewhere *different* than where you thought you would be at that point.

In John Maxwell's book *The 21 Irrefutable Laws of Leadership* he writes about what he calls "The Law of Process" (chapter 3).[224] He writes, "**What matters most is what you do day by day over the long haul...** What can you see when you look at a person's daily agenda? Priorities, passion, abilities, relationships, attitude, personal disciplines, vision, and influence. See what a person is doing every day, day after day, and you'll know who that person is and what he or she is becoming."[225]

> ... you should look at the overall destination of the path- over the long haul. And, you should work that process.

In other words, you should *not* bail out every time you see a bump. There are uphill climbs on *every* path. Rather, you should look at the overall destination of the path- over the long haul. And, you should work that process. I'm seeing that, regarding our Young Living business, if we learn the oils and use them, we're successful in our health and wholeness. We share that info with others- either because they ask or it arises naturally in conversations. They use the oils, then become intrigued and want to know more... and eventually order the kit.

---

[223] Ferriss has great points about working smarter rather than working harder, which he labels as being efficient and effective at the same time. That is, do the things that matter with intentionality. See Chapter 5, "The End of Time Management."

[224] See "The Law of Process," chapter 3 in *The 21 Irrefutable Laws of Leadership* by John Maxwell.

[225] See *The 21 Irrefutable Laws of Leadership*, pages 24-25. Emphasis added. Again, this links back to the idea we introduced in the beginning of this book: incremental change, over time, is exponential.

That particular road of learning and using and sharing leads to more people being blessed by the therapeutic properties of Young Living essential oils, more enrollments and a growing OGV and a growing business. It leads to more oils/products for us, it leads to larger paychecks, and it leads to a greater sense of abundance and financial stability.

Right road, but trouble on the road

If you've watched the movie *The Wizard of Oz*, you know that Dorothy travels down the Yellow Brick Road throughout the course of the film. Eventually, she finds herself in Oz- and meets the Wizard. Why does she end up in Oz? She ends up there *because that's where the road goes*- despite the trouble she encounters along the way. When Dorothy faced trouble- "lions, and tigers, and bears, oh my!"- she persisted. She set her face towards the yellow brick road *and kept marching.*

> ...the road still works- and it's most often a mistake to simply change paths, if we know the path we're on takes us to the intended destination...

In life, we often question the road we're on when the trouble comes. However, the road still works- and it's most often a mistake to simply change paths, if we know the path we're on takes us to the intended destination.[226] Think about that for a moment. If you're headed to the beach and get a flat tire, you don't change directions because you hit a minor setback! Yet people often do this very thing in "life." For instance:

- I see people in our ministry start stepping towards recovery and wholeness, meet a proverbial "flat tire" (i.e., lose a job, a friend bails out on them, something else upsetting happens), so they presume that the road was a bad road. They toss healing out the window.

- I've seen people start climbing their way out of debt, only to be hit with a surprise automobile breakdown. Instead of paying the bill and pressing on, they give up and go deeper into debt.

- I plateaued in my weight loss for about a week. I was eating right, I was exercising and even exercising harder when I couldn't drop

---

[226] Andy Stanley, *The Principle of the Path*, page 10f.

weight. About the fourth or fifth day I really thought about quitting altogether and just eating what I wanted. Thankfully, I didn't. I dropped two pounds in a single day- and continued down the road I wanted to travel.

Often, when we face the situations, we assume that the road we're traveling is the wrong road. It wasn't- it isn't. You just bumped into a pothole. Just re-align your wheels and keep going. **The road still goes where the road goes, regardless of the road hazards on the way.**

Pot hole on the drive to win

In January, Cristy's business was humming along great. She had 16 personal enrollments that month- in addition to the other enrollments throughout her team. She had a great paycheck (nice enough to payoff one of our girl's orthodontic work), and it looked like momentum was picking up. The next month, we boarded the plane to Hawaii- all expenses paid, courtesy of Young Living. Oddly enough, she had a *lower* paycheck that month. Her OGV moved up by the lowest margin it had ever moved. It looked like momentum was actually slowing down, virtually from one month to the next.

Amidst all of this, something strange happened. We were in Hawaii when her OGV bumped up just enough to move her to a new rank: Gold. The slight move happened on the last day of February, with about two hours left in the day. I remember it well, as it was the night we met in Gary's suite for dinner with the other Top Ten winners. This was the same evening her friend Fredia hit Silver, in part because Cristy helped her with a team promo at the last minute (and, in even *greater* part, to Fredia's consistent, diligent work).

Anyway, two days later we went online to Cristy's virtual office and discovered something odd- she had dropped *below* Gold. Her OGV fell by about 200pv or so, dropping her below the required volume to have achieved that rank! In other words, she achieved it- and then *unachieved* it overnight. People in our upline had already sent out congratulatory posts on FaceBook (with dozens of other people seeing and "liking" those messages). People in Hawaii were telling her their own version of "Congrats." Even Mary Young had hi-fived and hugged her while we were having that discussion about getting comfortable with multilevel marketing!

Cristy made several phones calls on the way home during our series of airport layovers. Finally, she was told the news: "Someone in your downline removed themselves from the organization… and that affected your OGV…"

And, of course, since she was barely over the Silver/Gold threshold, that removal (and the OGV that went with it) was enough to send us back to the lower rank. Then and there, in the Atlanta airport, I learned another Young Living lesson: you will likely have people who remove themselves from your downline for whatever reason. Don't sweat it. If they do, you guys probably weren't "jiving" well anyway. It doesn't mean they're "bad" and you're "good" anymore that it means they're "good" and you're "bad." Yes, it will sting and you'll be tempted to take it personally (especially if you drop rank!). We wanted to-especially knowing how much time a dear friend on our team had spent supporting, training, and trying to help the defector.

(An aside here: When people retreat from your organization, know this: they can move out from "under" you, but in doing so they lose their downline. In other words, they can't "pack up and move," they can only *move*.[227] Anybody they've sponsored stays where they are.)

> Just re-align your wheels and keep going. The road still goes where the road goes, regardless of the road hazards on the way.

Anyway, stuff like that makes you want to get bummed out. *Really*. Despite the fun you're having, despite the incredible people you're meeting on the journey, despite the money you are making, and despite what you've planned for the future. You might feel like throwing your hands in the air. You get frustrated for a bit, and then you remember… "Wow, I'm using really great products, things I would want to use *anyway*… I'm meeting all of these great people… I'm in Hawaii, of all places, because this incredible company has paid for me to come here…" And you come back to reality.

Then you realize that stuff like this *always* happens. It's just part of life:

- You will teach people about the oils and they will sign-up "under" someone else. You will meet with them, stay up late answering their

---

[227] Generally, they must have permission from the three people directly in their upline to move as well. Because this member was beyond their first 30 days of enrollment, I'm not sure how this happened without our knowledge in this case. Exceptions happen, I assume.

questions on text message, and even email them things you have researched for them. Then they'll go another direction.[228]

- You will go to teach a class, as Cristy has done, expecting fifteen or twenty people there. Two will show. And the host will be one of them. And that host might unintentionally refute everything you say, thereby making the class feel like a complete waste of time, and yet another night that you spent away from your family.

- You will strategically build someone's downline who wanted to grow the business, only to find out a few month's later that they don't have time for it…

- You will have months where "sign ups" are easy and come without much work, and then you will *toil* for weeks without much of anything.

Even while writing this book, we had our share of potholes. Well, in this example I'd consider it a sink hole! Did you know I wrote the next chapter of this book *twice?* It wasn't because I enjoyed doing it so much that I simply had to take a second run at it. Here's what happened:

I spent most of a Saturday putting the pieces of Chapter 7 together. The file saves on its own as you go. Pages, Apple's word processing app that I've been using to write the manuscript, kept crashing throughout the day. It would always reopen with the latest "save" intact. I didn't think much about it and kept working on the book at random intervals on Sunday. I even took it to a small conference that afternoon where I got a lot of great info to put in chapter 3, the one where we discussed essential oils in detail. That stuff never made the book, though, because that night I sat down to work for an hour or so after the kids went to bed. That's when I received another "crash" notice.

I went to open the file, as I'd done at least a dozen times throughout previous 24 hours and received the message "*Husbands field manual.pages* can't be opened." The file was there- I could even save it to a jump drive and place it on another computer. It just wouldn't open. It was *done*. Finished.

After a personal (and very demonstrative, might I add) meltdown, I resigned myself to the fact that the work from the previous day or so was gone, never to be retrieved again. So, I went to my latest back-up of my entire hard drive and

---

[228] The flip side is that, sooner or later, you'll find out that someone else taught someone about the oils and then they signed up under you.

had the version of the manuscript from three days earlier, limiting my losses to what I've described above.

I tell you this, though, I wanted to quit writing right then and there. I wanted to toss my computer out the window, honestly. I already had the testimonials from 6 of the 7 guys, I had the entire book outlined, I had 75% of everything written. But I hit a pothole / sink hole and I was done. But after a good night's rest, some prayer and encouragement, I woke up the next morning and started writing again. **In the end, the crash was nothing more than hitting a bit of trouble while traveling down the right road.**

When tough things happen, no matter how silly they are when you look at them in the rear-view mirror of life, make up your mind to simply stay on the road. Don't quit. You'll reach your destination. Why? *Because that's where the road goes*. Stay on it and, sooner than later, you'll arrive where you want to be.

Set your agenda, your goals. . .

The last morning we were in Hawaii, I went for a long run- and just *thought*. No running partner or conversation, no thinking through my "to do" list for the day ahead. Just empty space. And *silence*. Remember, to this point, I hadn't been involved in my wife's business.

> When tough things happen, no matter how silly they are when you look at them in the rear-view mirror of life, make up your mind to simply stay on the road. Don't quit...

At all. Other than wearing that t-shirt to her event and then editing that awesome video for her.

At some point, I just knew what I was going to do when we got back home. I had a tidy list that I actually looked forward to tackling.

My list looked like this:

☐ Write *this* book. This would have the two-fold purpose of helping me learn about the oils & the company Young Living, and then I'd be better prepared to assist in the business.

☐ Free up Cristy's time- up to two days a week where she can teach, train, get out of the house, or do whatever she needs to do. This meant I needed to make some adjustments at my office and back out of some projects where I was helping in a significant way.

- ☐ Begin attending the conferences and conventions with her, to educate myself and experience everything I could firsthand.

- ☐ Reevaluate the list and create another next step when the book is complete.

That list is different than the list other guys might show you. For instance, we have nine kids- so I don't always show up to a lot of her classes and assist. I stay close to home during those times. Perhaps that will change in the future as the kids get older.

As well, our pace is different than other people have. We've decided that Cristy will teach one class per week on most weeks, but no more than two. We know several people who teach two classes a day, two days a week, for a total of four classes per week. When they have sign-ups, it's always tempting for me to think, "Whoa! If we just stepped it up a notch, we could be doing so much better!" But, we prayed through the plan we made- and we were wise about what we could commit in light of all of our other commitments and our nine kids.

We also wrote down where we wanted to be in the company- and what that would look like. We defined what it would take to get there. As I'm writing this, our desire is for Cristy to reach Diamond. Yes, we want to go father than that- but this is the next best step for us. And there's a step (Platinum) we have to hit in between.

After writing down where we wanted to be, I built a roadmap from that destination to where we are now. We've decided to head in that specific direction, hitting the goals along the way, regardless of what pot holes we have to dodge (or roll through). It's the same way I planned my weight loss, to regain control of my health and well-being. I wrote the end result down, and began backtracking, building a map of how much weight I needed to lose each week, what foods I could and couldn't eat, and how often I would need to exercise. **In their words, I reverse-engineered these things.**

With the road map in hand for both my health and Cristy's business, I got to work. And **I did so at the pace we decided works for us.** Do you see that? We didn't let someone else choose our destination, for either issue. We decided. And I didn't let someone else dictate the pace. We did. Then we began taking the incremental steps in that direction with the pace we determined is best for us and our family.

I made spreadsheets and everything, and I began tracking the data. And I began watching my progress on the health side and her progress in the business. Once I defined things and began tracking them, it's almost like they became even more important and took on a life of their own. **Understanding the gap between where we are and where we want to be let us actually see what it will take to get there.** That way we can evaluate- with honesty- questions like these:

- Do we want to do this?

- What will it take to do it?

- Is the cost (of time, effort, energy) worth the payoff?

On days when we feel tired and Cristy has to rush out to teach a class, or during weeks when it seems we don't see each other for a few nights straight, we can relax knowing that we chose this path- and we chose it for specific reasons. It keeps us focused and keeps us from giving up in the middle of a busy season in which we are working on our dream.

We've decided that the short term cost is worth the long term gain.

Now, when we get to Diamond we'll re-evaluate. I'll draw another map, update my spreadsheets, and we'll take the next best steps for us. We'll evaluate the downlines and the OGV and the other factors and see what the next best steps are to get there. By the way, **there are other things we want to do, too.** Lately, I've had a conversation with my sister, Mandy, about building a "family leg" under my Mom & Dad- intentionally.

In our organization, Mandy is under Cristy, and my Mom is under Mandy. Mandy is one of our "Level 1" distributors. When Mandy signed up, Cristy thought about moving her somewhere, but the more she prayed about it, she really felt impressed to leave Mandy on her own. We think we can build Mandy's team with her help, that strategically places people under my Mom. Mom is on the Essential Rewards program which means she'll get a check for any commissions that are due to her.

> … we can relax knowing that we chose this path- and we chose it for specific reasons.

Can you imagine what difference it could make for my parents, both in their 60s, if I helped Mandy build her business by placing people under my Mom- even if my Mom didn't do much to help? We could set my parents up with a residual income that they've completely not expected. Honestly, my Dad did well in planning for retirement. He saved and invested since I was a kid- probably earlier than that. They'll be fine. But why should I leave them at "fine" if we have the ability to do something that makes them "better" than fine?

"No," for now, but not later

The "Oola guys" spoke the first full morning we were in Hawaii.[229] Dave told the incredible story about hitting his breaking point and realizing he needed balance in his life.[230] Then Troy grabbed a plate and a stick to illustrate the balance-issue.

He hoisted the plate sideways atop the stick and began twirling it, whirling it in a quick circle with the pencil brown stick. The plate would start to rise, then level… then wobble… then come back down. After a quick catch, he'd release it back on the stick… whirl, twirl… then level… then spinning quicker. He caught it, amidst some applause and cheers, then explained, "I've been working on that one awhile." Apparently, it was a *real* plate, because later Dave tossed it on the floor to demonstrate what it felt like when his life fell out of balance and was shattered.

Troy continued, "I was always impressed at the circus… whenever I saw a guy who spun these plates…" He described how the plate spinner would easily set two or three in motion before moving to the fourth and fifth…

"By the time he got to the fifth or so," Troy relayed, "the mood of the trick changed, though. At that point the spinner would have to make a decision: *Do I continue adding more plates, or do I make sure to keep what I've already got in the air without crashing…?*"

You've seen the gig. It turns into a comical madhouse. The guy runs back and forth like a chicken with its head cut off. He usually adds plates until they start loosing their speed, causing them to wobble, fall of the stick, and shatter on the floor.

"It's entertaining when it's part of a circus routine," Troy said, "but *it's not entertaining when it happens in your life…*"

---

[229] https://www.oolalife.com/faq#oolalife

[230] I'm not going to spoil it and tell you the story. Read the book.

Here's the truth: we all have a lot of plates that we're spinning, a lot of balls that we're juggling.

- Everybody can juggle one ball.

- Most people can juggle two.

- A few people can juggle three.

- Very few can juggle four or more.

The balls are like the plates. As long as you juggle what you can maintain, you're good. But once you over extend, you don't simply lose the ball- or the plate- or the priority- that you added at the end, you can lose *everything*. It's not just the final item, the one that was "one too many" that is gone. *Everything* falls.

This is where the *No-for-now-but-not-for-later* concept comes into play.[231] It simply acknowledges this: there are balls you want to juggle and plates you want to spin. But should you wait to spin some of them later instead of right now? In other words, **you give them a "No" for now, but that "No" doesn't last forever- you simply postpone the "Yes" for a future time.**

I'll give you a few examples of *No-for-now-but-not-for-later* at my house:

> It's not just the final item, the one that was "one too many" that is gone. Everything falls.

- Cristy and I would like a Land Rover LR3. A good used one will cost me about $10,000. That's not an expense we need to take on right now. We don't do debt and I don't have the cash available. One day we will. That car is a *No-for-now-but-not-for-later.*

- Last Fall I coached little league soccer- 5 of our boys (all of them that can walk!) played. This Spring, Cristy's business was picking up and our ministry was launching a thrift store. We decided to focus on those things. We didn't need to take anything else on. Soccer became a *No-for-now-but-not-for-later.*

- I'm trying to lose about 8 or so more pounds. White mochas, lattes, and snacks are a *No-for-now-but-not-for-later.* And, when I pick those drinks and snacks up again, I'll pick up *less* of them that I used to.

---

[231] I did not create this concept. I first heard it on the *Andy Stanley Leadership Podcast,* "Family Matters," January 3, 2014 episode. Go to 19:00 in the podcast for the concept. Go to https://itunes.apple.com/us/podcast/andy-stanley-leadership-podcast/id290055666?mt=2

- Cristy purposely slowed down *some* of her doula work.[232] Cristy has been doing this for almost a decade and is awesome at it. She's assisted with hundreds of births and receives phone calls and emails every week with people wanting her help at a birth. Right now, she's teaching more classes and holding more Young Living meetings, so she's taking less clients each month. It doesn't mean she's giving it up forever; it means that some of the potential clients are a *No-for-now-but-not-for-later.*

- She also postponed teaching some of her childbirth classes. She's an incredible speaker and is in demand as a childbirth educator. She's certified to do it. She's maintaining her certifications, but is not teaching during this season, even though she's always *loved* doing it. Why? Because teaching childbirth classes is a *No-for-now-but-not-for-later.*

- I've got manuscripts that need to be edited and books we've published at our nonprofit as part of the core curriculum for the program that we're ready to tweak and adjust. I love writing. It helps me really learn about a topic when I "focus in" and put my thoughts on paper. Why am I putting off something I really enjoy? Because it's a *No-for-now-but-not-for-later*.

- I'm working more from our house- as much as I can now. That way, Cristy can get out to go to meetings to help train other leaders or to plan events or to just get things done. Fortunately, I have the flexibility to work from home. Do I not like going to the office? Actually, I really enjoy it. We've got an incredible team of people that I get to work with. Being at the office for extended times is a *No-for-now-but-not-for-later* for me.

Do you see what I'm getting at? The things I'm saying "No" to right now are not bad things at all. But they are things I need to *not* pick up. By picking them up now, I compromise the other balls that I'm juggling, the other plates that I'm spinning. As such, we've started planning with the *No-for-now-but-not-for-later* mindset. We say "No" to a few things now, effectively focusing our energy on pushing the car for this season. **Those things are a "yes," just not a "yes" for right now. They are a "yes" for later.**

Remember the analogy Pastor James gave me from *The Four Year Career*? We've decided to spin the Young Living plate and get our business humming.

---

[232] A doula provides labor support and coaching for women during natural childbirth.

We'll spin those other plates in due time, because if we try to spin them all at the same time the odds are that they'll all collapse.

Face it: everybody is busy. I have a full-time job. Nine kids. A wife who was running this business *on her own* until I went to Hawaii with her. And all the other stuff that goes along with life.

You probably have your stuff, too. There are likely things you need to put off, just for now. You may even know what they are. You know, those things you really like (you may even love them). There's nothing wrong with them other than they occupy time that you could be investing in something else. And if you're like me, you don't need another thing to add, another plate to spin.

> There are likely things you need to put off, just for now.

So consider setting some other things down, even things you enjoy; not for forever, just for now. And don't set the things down that I set down- unless they're the things you've decided you should set down. Remember, it's your life, so you get to choose the destination, you get to choose the pace at which you travel, and you decide what happens now and what happens later.

Chart your course, get in your car and head towards your destination!

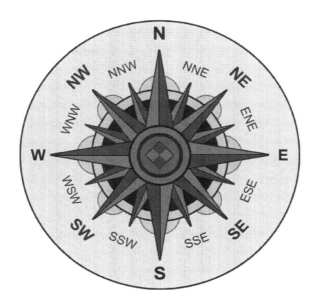

06: Direction: work it

Action steps

> **The main idea:** Your destination is determined by the direction you are headed. Decide where you want to go, plan your course, and start stepping in that direction.

☐ Define where you want to be in the company in 6 months. In a year.

☐ What is your "No, for now, but not for later" list?[233] What are the things you will stop doing- or postpone starting- so you can "push the car" for the next season?[234]

☐ 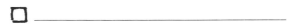 _____

---

[233] This might include Little League, Netflix, etc. Remember, these aren't "bad things." Some of the things you want to do (i.e., I want to train for an ultra-marathon) may be great. They're just not for now- they're for later.

[234] Warning: You might not need the libido podcast if you give your wife your list. On the other hand, you may need one that revives people who go into immediate cardiac arrest!

- ☐ _____
- ☐ _____
- ☐ _____

☐ "Reverse engineer" your way there. Write down the incremental steps it will take to arrive at that destination- no matter how small you think they are.

Want to know more?

☐ Read:

    ☐ "Dodging Bullets," Chapter 4 in Tim Ferriss' _The 4-Hour Workweek_

    ☐ "The End of Time Management," Chapter 5 in Tim Ferriss' _The 4-Hour Workweek_

☐ Listen:

    ☐ _Andy Stanley Leadership Podcast_, "Family Matters," January 3, 2014 episode. Go to 19:00 in the podcast for the _No-for-now-but-not-later_ concept.[235]

    ☐ To the relevant chapter of the audiobook

☐ Search:

    ☐ Search Oola's website (www.OolaLife.com). Notice how others are making progress forward towards their goals. See what you can learn and what ideas this may spark.

---

[235] https://itunes.apple.com/us/podcast/andy-stanley-leadership-podcast/id290055666?mt=2

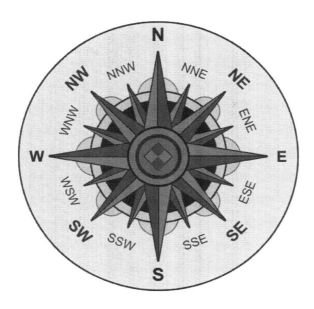

06: Together / Kent's story

We have always been an over-the-counter/prescription med-using family. All of that changed in October of 2012. And it all started with my chronic allergies. I have struggled with my allergies since I was a very small child. Growing up, I was on all sorts of prescription and over-the-counter allergy meds as well as daily allergy shots for seven years.

Kent Smith has been married to Stacy for 19 years. They have 3 teenagers and have been with Young Living since May 2013.

I grew tired of taking all of these meds and had gone off of them in my early adult life. In October of 2012, my dear wife, Stacy, was so tired of hearing me constantly clear my throat, that she begged me to go to the allergy specialist. I did. That is when things went terribly wrong.

Soon after the doctor visit, I started on the steroid nasal spray he'd prescribed me. I felt great for a couple of days, but then took a drastic turn.

To give my story the background that it needs for you to understand, I will let you in on what I do for a living. I work as a State Trooper for the State of Alabama in the Aviation Unit. I am a tactical flight officer, which means that it's my responsibility to guide the helicopter to its destination during rescue operations and criminal apprehensions. I operate the FLIR (forward looking infrared camera) in order to locate lost individuals or individuals fleeing/hiding from law enforcement.

We were conducting a huge training operation in October. When I say "huge", I mean HUGE! We had over 100 people on sight, including television and news media, State Emergency Management teams, and multiple high-angle rescue teams. They were all there to watch our demonstration on how to do a rescue extraction.

I was in my place in the back of the helicopter, making the calls as the crew chief, when all of a sudden, I began to feel strange things going on with my heart. I remember feeling like I was having heart palpitations and I was absolutely zapped of all energy. In fact, I almost couldn't pull the 100' rope back into the helicopter. This is a feat I've performed hundreds of times. I immediately notified the pilot to go back to the landing zone.

When we landed, the EMT's on site hooked me up to heart monitors. The readings all led to the same conclusion: I needed to get to the ER right then!

After many, many tests at the ER and cardiologist, it was determined, that I had PVC's. That was the only explanation for the way I had been feeling since I started the nasal spray - extreme fatigue, faintness, and the constant heart palpitations. The cardiologist could find no explanation why I had started having PVC's after a lifetime of being healthy. Stacy was very scared about what was happening to me. It was a very uncertain time for us. Stacy and I began brainstorming about what had changed in my life that might be attributing to this diagnosis. When we reflected, we realized the only thing that had changed was the use of the nasal spray. Stacy looked up that particular prescription on the Internet and there were so many reports of people experiencing PVC's as well as my other symptoms after using it.

The articles said that it would take six weeks for all of the medicine to get out of my system. I stopped taking it immediately. Because of my serious responsibilities at work (having other people's lives in my hands), I simply could not go back to work until all of my symptoms disappeared. This took four weeks. Four weeks of me being unable to get up and participate in normal, everyday life. I had no energy. It was a very tough time for our family.

Fast forward a few months later to allergy season of 2013. Stacy started seeing a dear friend of hers, Kelli Wright, posting about a natural remedy for allergies. For Stacy, this was a no brainer, and she told Kelli to "get us some of these, right away." She read a lot about the oils, as she loves to research and learn. Because she trusted Kelli, she ordered the Premium Starter Kit with my blessing. Though, I was very skeptical by the concept that essential oils could make a difference for my issues.

Now, fast forward again to almost a year later. I am a FULL believer in the power of these magnificent oils. We, as a family, haven't had to use any over-the-counter or prescription medicines since May of 2013. We are so thankful to God for the blessings of these oils and what they have done for our health. We are so grateful that our home is equipped, at all times, to treat various illnesses and issues that we face.

We have not been able to keep this good news to ourselves. We've been sharing the oils with everyone we know and many people that we don't know! God has blessed our business beyond what we could ever have imagined. He has blessed us financially and also spiritually in this journey. This is more than just a business. It is a ministry.

Is it always easy? Of course not! But, we know we're doing what God has called us to do, which is sharing alternatives to medicines and their sometimes (and often times) nasty side effects. It has been so much fun to partner together as a team, doing events together, educational classes together, conferences, and vendor booths. We have a story to share. We feel it is our responsibility to do so. And, we are having a blast doing it!

For those of you wondering how to support your wife in the "oil business", I would like to give you the things that I have learned:

1. Pray for her and the business.

2. Team with her and make it "y'all's" business.

3. Help her host classes, events, and work vendor booths.

4. Take time to sit down with her weekly, to discuss the schedule for the week and help her see ways that her time can be managed better.

5. Support her by rallying the family and getting the kiddos involved. For instance, as I am writing this, my three children are in the kitchen filling 300 bottles with carrier oil. There are so many ways to make this a family business. This pulls your family together even more.

6. Support her by listening, letting her bounce ideas off of you, and by taking up extra slack around the home.

It is my prayer that this is will be a joyous journey for you, as it has been for me. Get ready to be challenged and to grow!

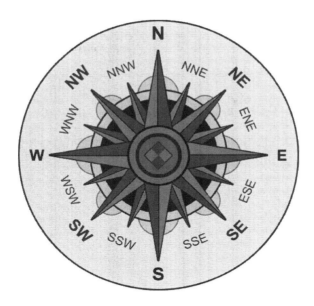

07: Raise the water level

A few years ago, when I was working at a church, I read an interesting point-of-view on "church growth." The author of the book *Natural Church Development*, Christian Schwarz, said that all growing churches have eight characteristics in common. His list isn't relevant to our conversation here: the way he puts the concepts together is, however. You see, Schwarz likened each trait to a slat on a bucket. Basically, they are the slats that form a container in which something can be held (in this case, people). In order for the church to grow, he said, an existing congregation didn't necessarily have to grow to a 100% in all of these areas, they could work on one at a time, choosing to raise the level of the weakest slat.

> **The main idea:** You don't have to master everything at once. Just improve one thing, and the water level rises for everything else.

The lowest slat, he said, was creating the point of exit. And, just as water will leak from the lowest hole in a bucket, so also would people "leak" from the lowest needed trait. In other words, he was saying that you can have inspiring worship services (trait #5) but if you do not have loving relationships (trait #8), the church will not grow. If you raise the weakest slat, however, you raise the level... and you can hold more people. Hang on to this mental image- we'll come back to it.

People who are a lot smarter than I am say you can apply the same theory to organizations- like nonprofits where I work and businesses where you may work. The slats will all be different, but they're there. When one of them is low, that becomes your point of exit. In the same way that a chain is only as strong as its weakest link, **a bucket can only hold water to the height of the lowest slat on the bucket.**

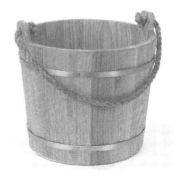

I saw this happen at my workplace a few years ago. We have an incredible team now- but we've had a long, hard road getting the team who, now, fits together beautifully. For an extended season, we had a great set of individuals (all great people), but we weren't a great team. In our case, we had a high slat for "mission"- *who doesn't want to see lives changed, people set free from addictions, and families reunited?* However, we had a low slat on "unity." Everyone really wanted to do their own thing (all good things), and we all felt constantly pulled in different directions. As a result, some valuable, smart people began leaving... slowly, but steadily.

Buckets and bicycles, slats and spokes

So, back to the Oola guys (you know, Troy, who spun the plate and then Dave smashed it on the floor...)[236] One of their chief ideas is that life must be lived in balance- that you can't throw yourself "all in" to any single area or things get out of whack.

They say a well-balanced life includes the following seven areas:

- Fitness

- Finance

---

[236] www.oolalife.com

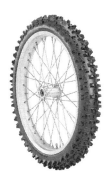

- Family

- Friends

- Field (your career / work)

- Faith

- Fun

Those areas look good to me. If I was going to even make a guess as to what slats would create a "life bucket" I don't think I could do any better than that. They seem to nail it down. These areas must all be balanced, the guys say. They suggest you visualize a wheel- like you have on your bike. They argued convincingly that each of the seven areas of life is a single spoke. In order for the wheel to turn, you need all of them. Lose one, you may be alright- for a while. Lose half of them and the wheel won't roll at all.

Change metaphors back to the bucket, again. Consider the seven "Oola areas" as your slats. *How much water can you hold?* If you're all work and no play (read: all "field" and no "fun"), how much water do you think you can hold? If you're faith quotient is high, but you don't

> *The main idea:* You don't have to master everything at once. Just improve one thing, and the water level rises for everything else.

have any friends… is that enough? If you're like me, some of the slats rank higher than the others. Or, to use their mental image, some spokes don't make it from the rim to the hub.

Right now, life may be so frustrating that you may think you need to change *everything* in order to move closer to your dreams. That's simply not true. All you need to do is find out what your weakest / lowest "slat" is… and then work to raise the water level in your "personal bucket." Then keep raising from there.

Think about it like this:

- You can take care of your personal fitness, now. Yes, you may need a bit of time- and a series of incremental steps- to hit your goal. But I've found that **starting is the hardest part. It's easy to continue** *once you've begun*. Consider that slat raised. Now, the water level is getting higher.

- You can take care of the finance part- or at least start moving in that direction- *if you just put some things on paper*. That helps a lot. Watch the level rise.

- If you've been following half of the advice I've given you in this book, you've probably already surrounded yourself with some great men. I'm not knocking your old friends- or even saying that you need to get rid of them. Ever. But *having some people who are moving in the same direction you are- with the same goals and encouraging you along the way- is massive*. The water level is getting higher.

- You're probably taking the idea of your family seriously- and even your "field" (or your wife's, which is *also* yours now) if you've made it this far. Do you see it? The water level is up…

Vote yourself most likely to succeed

One of the greatest myths circulating is that the person with the best education, most skills, and greatest amount of experience will be the most successful. They'll have the highest slats all the way around their bucket. And their spokes will all work right.[237] This is simply not true. There are *multiple* factors involved in determining who will be successful.

I asked a few distributors who were on the trip with us in Hawaii how they were allocating the money they were now making. Some of them were making *sizable* checks- as in more income in a month than they used to make in an entire year.

"Paying off debt," most of them said. I heard it *repeatedly* in various renditions throughout the entire trip.

Several of them talked about failed businesses, even failed stints with MLMs. A handful said they trusted the wrong business partners and had significant amounts of money stolen from them. One couple trusted the payroll company to

---

[237] See Dan Miller, *48 Days to the Work You Love*, pages 95-96.

pay the income taxes for their entire business' payroll each quarter, but the payroll service paid *themselves* instead! Two or three had lost jobs and were out of work right about the time their essential oil businesses started growing. I don't know that I met more than a few people on that trip who had been what the world would consider "successful" before they succeeded working the business side of Young Living.

Most of them were average. They were people like you and me, living paycheck to paycheck. Some of them wondered where the next meal might come from. And these are incredible people. They are humble. Gracious. Generous. Radically hospitable and loving. *And they are all persistent.*

Mary Young portrayed herself the same way the first time Cristy and I met her after a dinner party in Hawaii. She's an MLM rockstar, now, but she told us about how things used to be…

> I don't know that I met more than a few people on that trip who had been what the world would consider "successful" before they succeeded working the business side of Young Living.

"I was so in debt," she told us. "In fact, my entire family was in debt. We were all drowning in it."

Mary succeeded at her first networking marketing business- as a distributor, not an owner. Yes, she started at the bottom, just like each one of us.

"The first thing I did was start paying off those debts," she said. "Mine and then… one by one… one right after the other… I started getting my family free of the bondage they had been in, too." She smiled and spoke with a rushed excitement as she relayed the story. You could tell it was one of those pivotal moments in her life, as memorable as Gary's story about the French distiller.

Mary talked about her experience of "doing MLM" before you could go online and check your stats, too: "We had to wait each month until the fax came in. You'd look at it and it would tell you what everyone was doing… Nothing like we have now."

As she said that, I wondered about all the Diamonds, Crown Diamonds and Royal Crown Diamonds and other people above us in Young Living who had paved the way for us to succeed quickly, because they had been persistent and willing to succeed intentionally and deliberately. I thought about what that must have been like.

Mary told us that she did buy a car. As she knocked off the debt she made one significant purchase.

"I had been driving an old beat-up Volkswagen," she laughed. Her face lit up as she explained that she would "park it way away from the crowds- where nobody could see what I drove to the meetings."

She learned that she was eligible for a car when she hit a certain rank with this other MLM, so she went for it. She made it, then got the best vehicle that the car allowance would furnish, a brand-spanking new Mercedes Benz.

Now, lest you think she went all flashy with the first bit of success, let me let you in on the buzz from a few friends who have been to Gary and Mary's house: apparently *the same* Mercedes still sits in the garage today! I knew the Young's were genuine and sincere the moment I met them. I hear tales like this that come in small bits and pieces from random distributors who interact with them, each of them confirming what I already sense to be true.

If I can do this, anybody can. . .

I sat next to Jeremiah during breakfast one morning. His wife, Monique, has shattered every record and every time line that's ever existed for Young Living Distributors. I mentioned that a few pages back. When I met him, he had just resigned from what he considered a dream job in order to assist her.

"I tell you," he said, "if I can do this… if we can do this… anybody can." Then- "I'm not that smart for things to be going as well as they are."

Let me clarify, Jeremiah *is that smart*. He is a tech guy who could probably do anything he wants to do, but he wasn't walking in false humility that morning. He was getting at something like this: **the success we've had is far superior to what we even thought possible.**

Jeremiah explained to me that Monique has a unique way of seeing trends and reading culture and interacting with people. He's dead on. She does. He told me that she used to know what to buy in advance when they had a scrapbooking business, back when that was the "in" thing. She always knew ahead of the curve what everyone would want.

"She would pick the right colors, the right designs… I was always surprised at how well it worked…"

We talked about FaceBook and how he helps with the family business. We spoke about how the Lord opened the door for him to walk out of a job that he thought he would never leave. And he never would have, if the conditions hadn't been undeniably mind-blowing.

"We were able to buy a car recently," he told me. "A Jeep."

It was what they had wanted for a while. The back story to the Jeep is that they used to be a one-car family. Apparently, the key was stuck in the ignition of the old Forerunner, so they just left it unlocked. They air didn't work, either, so they had to drive fast with the windows down to get cool in the summer and had to bundle up and get warm in the house before riding in the winter.

Apparently, Monique made it to the local Jeep dealership before Jeremiah that day. She was ready to pay the sticker price before he got there, and thought he was being rude when he tried to haggle. "The price was there for everyone to see," Monique says. "I thought you just pay the price that's there- just like at other stores!"

> He was getting at something like this: the success we've had is far superior to what we even thought possible.

We all laughed.

Then I asked Jeremiah if he paid cash for it, if he walked into the dealership, stroked a check, and walked out with the keys to a brand new automobile in his hand. In turn, he told me something that confirmed what I already believed: he was smarter and more persistent than he let on.

"No. Not yet. Not time for that yet," he said with a grin. Then, "That will come. Right now, we're paying off debt." He shared that they don't have the scrapbook business anymore, and are now able to pay the debts they owe from it. He explained that a year ago they were "flat broke" (his exact words). They borrowed gas money to get home from his sister's wedding almost one year ago to the day that we sat there eating breakfast.

"A lot has changed in a year," he laughed. *"A whole lot."*

You see, he's down-to-earth just like the rest of us. *Perhaps, their story even hits close to home?* Furthermore, I'm betting that if you had a line up on the exact day that Jeremiah and Monique enrolled as distributors you might not have picked them to smash every record in Young Living history. Sure, you can talk them for just a few minutes and tell that they've got the tenacity to succeed. But the ability to smash the record books?

What happened? Two incredible people graciously continued putting one foot ahead of the other, helping countless others, and leaving a wake of healing and health and hope behind them. And they're still going.

It's not perfect people who succeed. Rather, it's humble people who are persistent. It's people who are honest and sincere, who share their successes (Jeremiah showed me income projections and spreadsheets and taught me a lot in a few conversations) and share their failures (how's his story for genuine transparency?).

By the way, this year they started a new family tradition. This Christmas they went to IHOP, each of them taking $100 with them. They prayed over their envelopes in which they placed the money and asked the Lord to lead them to the right person to give it to. The stories they tell from the experience are tear-jerkers. Every single one of them.

The "Outliers"

A study at Yale University reported the following:

- 15% of a person's success is due to education, skills, and experience.

- 85% is due to interpersonal skills- including attitude, enthusiasm, self-discipline, desire, and ambition.

Do you see something strange from that list? The things we typically attribute to success- things like education and experience- aren't indicators at all. After listening to the stories of mountain-sized debt, failed business, and trusting the wrong people, I've seen living proof. **The people who succeed are the ones who will not be denied success.** They keep pushing and pushing until a door opens for them.

I have friends with law degrees working in fast food restaurants; I have friends with no college experience serving in large ministries or running successful business ventures. In my own organization I have people with impressive resumes, and I have people with large gaps in their resumes reflecting when they were incarcerated for years- even decades. Both groups serve at every level in the organization.

Many times, the person who looks best "on paper" doesn't get the job. Why? Because, sometimes, people who look good on paper (i.e., they have a very "high slat" in the area of "field" or "finance") also have a low

> It's not perfect people who succeed. Rather, it's humble people who are persistent.

slat that is leaking somewhere else. Maybe their personality is haughty or they have a sloppy personal presentation. Or maybe they're just not fun at all.

In their book, *Oola,* Troy and Dave quote actor Will Smith:

> *The only thing that I see that is distinctly different about me is I'm not afraid to die on a treadmill. I will run. I will not be outworked, period! You might have more talent than me, you might be smarter than me, you might be sexier than me, you might be all of those things. You got it on me in nine categories. But if we get on the treadmill together, there's two things: You're getting off first, or I'm going to die! It's really that simple.[238]*

You see, most success simply comes down to the person who decides to put one foot in front of the other consistently over the long haul. Think incremental change. Lots of it. Over the long haul.

Malcolm Gladwell is a story-telling sociologist who has written a book entitled *Outliers*. In that book he notes that much of the success we see in others and

---

[238] *Oola*, Kindle Location 1695-1698.

attribute to "talent" or "luck" or "right place at the right time" is simply hard work that suddenly manifests and is visible seemingly overnight.

He argues that Bill Gates, for instance, didn't become an overnight success in the computer industry when he created Microsoft and then later launched Windows. Rather, Bill Gates grew steadily towards success through hours and hours of learning programming by working on a large main-frame computer at a nearby college campus. He spent countless nights in front of the screen from the time he was young, until we all finally saw his "instant" fame and fortune.

Gladwell writes about Olympians and world-class violin players in the same way. We marvel at what they do and speak about how they are "gifted" and "unique." Without detracting from them in the slightest, Gladwell says they are "outliers"- meaning their skill sets and abilities lie outside the normal bounds of what is average, because they spend so much time preparing and training.

Specifically, he says that something happens at the 10,000 hour mark- *that* particular amount of time and attention given to anything makes someone an expert in it. If you dance for 10,000 hours you're going to be amazing. If you teach for 10,000 hours, you're going to learn

> ...most success simply comes down to the person that decides to put one foot in front of the other consistently over the long haul. Think incremental change. Lots of it. Over the long haul.

something about the craft of public speaking and integrate it into your delivery so much so that you excel. If you run for 10,000 hours you are going to be fast and strong. In other words, **the people who stand out are, at the end of the day, the people who persist.** They are the ones who choose to put one foot in front of the other over the long haul.

By the way, I read an interesting stat in *The Four Year Career*. The author suggests that if you invest 2 hours a day, for 6 days a week, for 50 weeks a year... in four years you will achieve, you guessed it, 10,000 hours. You'll be an expert.[239] If you want to be an expert at Young Living faster, re-run the math and set your course. Then persist.

---

[239] This idea was cited in *The Four Year career,* Kindle location 283.

The big rocks

Back in my seminary days, I was assigned Stephen Covey's book *The Seven Habits of Highly Effective People* for a leadership class. That book outlined some principles I've relayed to you over the past few pages. For example, Covey says you should "begin with the end in mind."[240] Reverse engineering your life is doing just that. He also says you think "win-win" instead of "win-lose."[241] And, relevant to our discussion here, he teaches that you should put "first things first."[242]

I love how he illustrates this last one- *putting first things first.* He set a pitcher on a table and then sets a few large rocks beside it. They're chunky, but small enough to fit in the clear container next to them. Then he sets a pile of pebbles next to the rocks.

"Will it all fit it?" he asks.

He begins setting the small pebbles inside the pitcher and they reach the halfway point. It becomes obvious that there's too much on the table to fit into that pitcher without forcing it all in and shattering the container.

Finally, he stops and says something like, "What if we do it like this…?"

> The only difference is the order in which things went into the pitcher. *Or into your bucket.* Nothing more.

Then he dumps the pebbles out and sets the large rocks in *first*. They all fit. Then he begins dropping pebbles in. They fall through the gaps between the rocks, find their way to the lowest point in the clear pitcher and settle. Other pebbles fall on top of them. In the end, everything fits and the pitcher isn't even full.

He then asks, "What made the difference?" The only difference is the order in which things went into the pitcher. *Or into your bucket.* Nothing more. I suppose you see the bigger picture now, in some sense. There are slats, spokes, and rocks in your own life. They're all the same, regardless of the imagery you use.

---

[240] Habit 2, Begin with the end in mind, teaches this concept.

[241] Habit 4

[242] Habit 3

The point, here, is that you know what those important items are for you- and you that begin living them with intentionality.

The weekly review

Here's one thing I've learned about these big rocks. They must be *scheduled*, or they simply will not happen. Other things- less important things- will creep in and take their place. Before long, your day will be full and you'll find yourself out of time with little pieces of metal (instead of spokes), random pieces of wood (instead of a slat), and plenty of things still left to do (you'll have a handful of rocks you're still carrying around in your pocket).[243]

That's where the idea of The Weekly Review comes into play.[244] Every week, you should set aside at least 1-2 hours to take inventory of the previous week, as well as make plans for the upcoming week. The short amount of time you spend in the review will multiply itself in terms of productivity as you persist through your week, systematically taking the next best steps for you and your family.

Here is what I do during my weekly review, which I currently do every Sunday afternoons while my youngest kids are napping and my oldest ones are jumping on the trampoline:

- #1- File all loose papers

- #2- Review the previous week's calendar

- #3- Preview the next week's calendar- and, often, the week after that.

- #4- Identify the big rocks for the week.

- #5- Look at what I delegated to others last week.

- #6- Evaluate what I want to read / study this week.

---

[243] Remember the "No, for now, but not forever" issues that you've already decided.

[244] This concept comes from Michael Hyatt's e-Book, *Life Plan*, page 33f.

- #7- Write it down

#1- File all loose papers

The first thing I do after sitting at the dining room table is empty my wallet of receipts. I take every piece of paper from my backpack, and I look through my notebook. I place the receipts in my expense log. I either file, scan, or throw away *all* loose papers. It's my way of decluttering.

Throughout the week, Cristy hands me all of her receipts from lunch appointments, business meetings, and even provides me with the addresses where she taught classes and or meetings. I scan her receipts into my computer, log everything into a spreadsheet, and file the hard

> ...these big rocks... must be *scheduled*, or they simply will not happen. Other things- less important things- will creep in and taken their place.

copies in case of a lovely IRS audit. I don't worry about doing this stuff every night when she hands those pieces of paper to me- I know that I have a designated time where I'll eventually get to it.

As well, I used to keep all of my notes from various office meetings in a separate folder for each project I was managing. This meant that, often, I was carrying around 8-10 folders. Now, I use *one* notebook. I take it to meetings and carry it with me to write notes when I study. *Everything* goes in it- so I always know where everything handwritten is located. It's either in that notebook or it doesn't exist. At the end of the week, I review the notes. I take out what I can and scan it into my computer. Then I toss the hand-written sheets away. It's the system that currently works for me.

You may thinking, right now, that you don't have that many sheets of loose paper. I guarantee you have *more* than you think. You may have lists of things you meant to do, sheets with stuff you are learning about the oils, and even notes you've taken while pushing your way through this book. You may have a few pay-stubs. If you've gone to any Young Living events with your wife, you have marketing pieces, info about the compensation plan, and other random items. Toss some of it in the trash, and file what you want to keep.

Once you start working on a system to get/stay organized, it will free your mind to focus on your family when you're home, versus feeling scattered and pulled in a bunch of different directions. My suggestion is to get a few folders and keep them in a single filing cabinet so that you know where everything is stored. Then you can find it later. Sort them by topic, so you have everything handy. Throw everything else away.

#2- Review the previous week's calendar

After decluttering, I look back to see what I left undone that was on my calendar. The fact is that, each week, a large portion of my "to do" list simply gets pushed to the following week. I used to sweat it. Now, I don't. It just is what it is. That's where I'm at in life right now. There are often phone calls I wanted to make and emails I wanted to send that I simply did not have time to do. I make note of those on the following week's calendar.

If I can handle the undone task in less than two minutes, I actually do it *right then.* That means I will go ahead and send an email or even make a phone call to someone's office- even on Sunday afternoon. My logic is that it will take me about half that time to write it in my calendar and push it off, and by handling it right then I put the burden on them to call me back rather than me chasing them down during my week.

This propensity towards action, rather than procrastination, seems to work well for me. Unless It's something related to laundry: washing, drying, folding, putting away. Then, I tend to lean towards procrastination. Did I mention my wife is editing this book? She may or may not have added that part.

In addition to phone calls and emails that didn't get done, I also look at meetings that had to be rescheduled- whether I postponed them or the other person did. If it was important enough for me to calendar the first time, I check to see what the status is. Many times the issues I needed to meet about simply resolve themselves without a meeting; sometimes they don't. But I want to take the time and find out where things are.

For you, this may mean looking back at projects you needed to complete or other opportunities you just needed to evaluate. It may also mean that you need to look at how many hours you worked, so that you know what kind of paycheck to be expecting the following week- particularly if you are an hourly employee.

You'll want to know how this effects your finances in light of your wife's work in her essential oil business. That means you'll probably want to look at her virtual office. Find out what changed from the previous week.

Finally, you may have things to do for her, things you committed to do in order to help her grow the business. You're saying "No, for now, but not for later" to a few things so that you can push the car up the hill. See what got done and what didn't. Make sure you are persisting at the right priorities, that you are raising slats and placing spokes- not just tinkering with wood chips and chunks of metal.

#3- Preview the next week's calendar- and, often, the week after that

In Step #2 I primarily looked *back* at the previous seven days; in Step #3 I look *forward* to the next seven. I take a 30,000 foot view of the new week, looking at it from high above. This *always* gives me a different perspective than I have once I'm in the middle of the actual hustle of the week itself.

> Once you start working on a system to get/stay organized, it will free your mind to focus on your family when you're home, versus feeling scattered and pulled in a bunch of different directions.

At this point, before the week begins, I'm merely looking at what's on the agenda. I can see what meetings I have, what days I can set aside to catch up on writing, and evaluate ongoing projects that I need to push a few yards down the field. Many times, looking at the week before it begins actually highlights things I need to adjust.

For instance, a few weeks ago I had a long workout scheduled the same day that we planned to be at a Young Living conference. I knew there was no way I could do the longer workout *and* make it to the event on time, without getting up extremely early. So, I swapped the short workout from another day with the long workout on that day and things went smoothly.

I particularly review Cristy's teaching schedule and note if she has any classes on the docket (most weeks, yes), if we've made dinner plans with any other couples (about two times a month), and see if I'm on dock to either keep the kids or secure a babysitter. I find it helpful to look ahead *now* rather than finding myself sinking just a few days later.

Usually, I look at the following few weeks during this time, as well. We often have a few lingering things that can sneak up fast. Travel schedules. Conferences and larger events. Projects that have deadlines two or three weeks out but need a big dent put in them now.

Here's why looking ahead is important for me: I've got so much going on that if you tell me something and I don't write it down, I'll probably forget it. So, if it's important, I write it down. If I'm supposed to do something for you, I write it down. If you're supposed to do something for me, I write that down, too. *Then I can forget about it.* I do this with meetings, too. When I think of topics I want to discuss at a staff meeting, I simply write it down in the notes section of my calendar and forget about it. The info is there for me when I'm on my way to the meeting in which I'll discuss it. I just have to remember to check my calendar-the one place where I keep everything. And that happens easiest if I have a set time when I review it.

Keep each of your similar items on your calendar, too, and they will never catch you by surprise... as long as you have a set time at which you review the calendar! For example: Keep all of your meeting notes in one place, all of your "to do" lists in one place, etc. There's nothing worse than missing something important- and only remembering when you see it in a calendar that you forgot to check![245]

#4- Identify the big rocks for the week

Each week, I evaluate the list of "big rocks" I've got.[246] I'm not changing the rocks at this time; I am insuring that there are action steps associated with each, and that the activities are actually making forward progress. I've discovered that

---

[245] I use a MacBook Air. It syncs with my iPhone and my iPad Mini. Find a system that works for you.

[246] http://andrewejenkins.wordpress.com/2011/10/24/big-rocks-first/

if you do not have an action step for a priority, as well as have a time set aside for that priority, then it is not really a priority- it's just an intention, a desire, a dream, or a wish.

This part of my weekly review doesn't take too long, because **many of these items are scheduled the same from week to week**. For instance, I know that I will always drive my oldest girls to gymnastics and dance on Monday afternoons. I do specific things with the boys at other dedicated times. I know that Cristy and I will almost always have a date night on Wednesday evenings. I workout at 6:30 am each morning. I meet a few of the guys from church every Tuesday morning at 9:00. I've set each of these items on the "repeat" function in my calendar. If you look six months out, they're already there- nothing gets scheduled on top of them.

> I've got so much going on that if you tell me something and I don't write it down, I'll probably forget it. So, if it's important, I write it down.

Your life is going to change. Growth *always* brings change. One of Oola's core statements is "balance and grow." If I heard it once, I heard it seventeen times. Balance and grow, balance and grow, *balance and grow…* "Balance and grow" means that you keep your priorities in order- all of them. You don't neglect any to the exclusion of the others. If you do that, and you'll get a flat tire. Or the water will start flowing out of your bucket instead of into it. You *want* change, and you *want* growth. Not just *balance*, that we so often find ourselves saying we need.. **Everything that's dead is in perfect balance. But it's not growing. It's not alive.** Get ready for change. It's certain. You will have a growing home-based business, you will have a network of new friends, and you will have some financial decisions to make. Your action steps will likely change, too.

Amidst all of this change, though, notice that the purpose of the weekly review is not to continue identifying and re-identifying priorities (i.e., rocks, spokes, slats). That's already been done. At this point you're looking at implementing your priorities, not discovering them. You're intentionally setting aside time to chart the growth, ensuring that it aligns with where you've decided to go.

I currently use the "Oola seven" as my big rocks. After hearing Troy and Dave speak, I knew they were putting better language to something I'd been putting together for awhile. I've placed my current list below- the things I strive to do each week. You'll notice that some of the areas have less information than the others. That means that those slats are currently low or that those spokes need some adjustment. No worries, though, since I have things written down it's much easier to get an honest picture of where things are and move them to where I want them to be in due time.

Big rocks need action steps

Big rock	Action step	Why it matters
Fitness	Exercise 6 days a week, currently using Insanity's T25 program Nutrition- monitor what I eat and when	I currently write both of these items in a spreadsheet each day, along with tracking my weight. I find I'm more conscientious and consistent when I can see it on paper.
Finance	Manage business spreadsheets for Cristy's essential oil business Oversee the teams at my office responsible for financial income to the nonprofit (this could be with "field" as well), but since we started the organization these things seem so intertwined right now- and b/c out income is directly tied to this	This lets us see where we are on "the plan" we've created, and keeps us focused on not moving too quickly- but pacing ourselves Things get really stressful when we operate out of our means- or don't keep spending in check
Family	Wife- Wednesday Date Night Kids- Spend one-on-one time with each kid every week / do something fun as a group at least once a week	This helps us remove ourselves from everything else- including the rest of the family- and reconnect We have a lot of kids- it's important to have specific things (even if small) that I do with each
Friends	Pull away from the office with one of the guys on staff each week Take time each week to meet with one of the guys, not on staff, who is a friend	These are some of my best friends- so we pull away from the office, even if we end up talking shop some of the time (even better if we do something not related to work at all) Spontaneous stuff is great- but most people have too much going to just be spontaneous- schedule the time

Big rock	Action step	Why it matters
Field	Keep focused on the things at work that only I can do	This keeps be from getting bogged down with things other can do better- and should be doing- lest I edge them out of their own "sweet spot"
	Other items as scheduled	Most of the things I do each week have placed as standing appointments (whether it's updating my blog, returning emails, writing grants, etc.)
Faith	Worship each Sunday, read my Bible and pray during the week	This keeps me aware of my connection to our Father
	Make time to simply clear my mind and reflect…	Each day, I get alone with my Father. I read, I pray. I listen to Him and to some great music. Weekly, I use my Sunday afternoon long run to think and pray over my priorities for the upcoming week… before my review. It awakes me, rather than puts me in a nap-like state, and my mind really connects with the upcoming week while I'm away from the phone, the computer, and everyone else.
Fun	Schedule something with my wife and kids each week	Sometimes these are bigger things (trips), sometimes they are small (like sneaking out on a weeknight for coffee)

#5- Delegated to others

I work in an office overseeing a growing group of people. I regularly delegate tasks to them. The same is true with volunteers who handle projects for our ministry. While I'm looking at what's behind me and what's ahead, I also look at the running list I keep of things that have been delegated to others. By the way, I keep this list- and all other lists- in the "Reminders" app on my iPhone. That way it updates to my laptop and my iPad. If I put it in one place, I have it everywhere.

Sometimes I've delegated things as small as making me a set of keys for something.[247] Other times, I've empowered someone to do something like set a meeting with other ministry leaders and their teams. We find ourselves dealing with real estate issues, grant projects, and writing projects. I do *not* worry about these issues all week- I review them once a week and follow-up. Sometimes this means I send an email *right then* to get a status update.

If you're not "the boss" at work, you may think you don't have things that you've delegated. I guarantee you have delegated far more than you might realize. Consider the following:

> I've discovered that if you do not have an action step for a priority, as well as have a time set aside for that priority, then it is not really a priority- it's just an intention, a desire, a dream, or a wish.

- Was a prospective client supposed to call you back? Then you have delegated a phone call. It may be time to follow-up with them.

- Was someone in your downline supposed to get with you about setting up a class? You've delegated a calendaring item.

- Was someone in your upline supposed to help you with something? You've delegated a task.

Write each of these down the first time you delegate them- then forget about them. Leave it in the hands of the person you appointed for the task. Just be sure you check your list once a week. Because you might need to follow-up.

#6- Evaluate what I want to read / study

Instead of trying to read a few books at the same time (which is what I used to try to do), I focus on one. At the beginning of the week, I decide what I'm reading that week. I try not to do any other "impulse reading", including grabbing random magazines at the check out line and mindlessly surfing the

---

[247] I intentionally don't have a a key to our main facility or our thrift store, and use a keypad on my door. The key is one less thing to deal with. Sometimes, I find I do actually need a key, though.

Internet. It's a trap for me that eats away time like nothing else. Plus, I'm mentally sharper when my mind is not garbled with so much clutter.

On a side note, I don't read the newspaper and I don't watch the evening news. On one hand, I know that sounds irresponsible; on the other, if something incredibly important happens in the world, I'll hear about it from everybody else on their FaceBook feed or while I'm sitting at the coffee shop. I can then intentionally research and study more about what I want to know about. I know, I miss a lot of breaking news this way- I never hear about the latest thing that happened first. But I have no control over what breaks and what happens after it breaks, anyway. So why fill my mental space with it?

> I simply write it down... forget about it. The info is there for me...

Here's another tidbit: Some weeks I don't read anything at all. If I've been particularly bogged down in something, I mentally take it easy for a week or two. I find that I'm sharper and quicker when I get back on it.

#7- Write it down

Back in the day, when I was using a Franklin Covey planner, I used the "two pages per day" version. Every day had a left page and a right page. The left had a timeline for the day, running from top to bottom; the right page was blank for notes. I vividly remember making a list of phone calls and emails that I needed to handle on each page, *every single day.* Most of the time, the list just got shifted from one day to the next. That meant I spent a lot time each day just reorganizing my "to do" list, and it meant I was re-doing the same thing virtually.every.single.day. It was grossly inefficient.

As I mentioned earlier, I currently enter everything into my iPhone *or* MacBook Air *or* iPad Mini, and the events sync from one to the other wirelessly. If it's in one place, it's everywhere. That means my notes for meetings and even my contacts are on each device. It makes staying organized much simpler.

In addition to the electronic calendar and notes, I also have a few headings on a single sheet of paper:

- **Calls.** These are people I need to call during the week. Rather than putting this down for a particular day, I just try to get it done sometime that week. If it has to happen a specific time, I calendar it like any face-to-face meeting.

- **Emails.** Same as calls. I usually make a short note of what the email is about. If I can handle actually sending that email in 2 minutes or less, I don't put in on my list- I just go ahead and send it right then.

- **To do.** This may include errands I need to run, letters I need to write (thank you letters to donors, or letters of recommendation for people completing the program at the nonprofit, etc.).

- **Other.** Sometimes I have something that defies categorization. It's not a phone call, an email, or even something to do. It goes here.

I realize that I could probably keep this list on my electronic devices, too. I just haven't found a way that works for me consistently well. And, for me, there's something about scratching things off a list that is more satisfying than simply pressing the "delete" button on a computer.

Do your thing, not mine

I placed a simple diagram on the next page to show you how this all fits together for me. You'll notice that the 7 Rocks, Spokes, & Slats come from this chapter. They're the Oola list. The 7 Ways to Grow Your Young Living Field were found in Chapter 5 of this book, "Getting traction." There we discussed practical things you can do right now to help your wife succeed. The Weekly Review list melds what I've just described above.

That's my current system. It's what works for me now. My guess is that some of it will work for you and some of it won't. How you plan and implement your priorities is not as important as the fact that you actually do it. Use trial and error, and find a system that works for you.

The Weekly Review

7 Rocks, Spokes, & Slats

Fitness

Finance

Family

Friends

Field

Faith

Fun

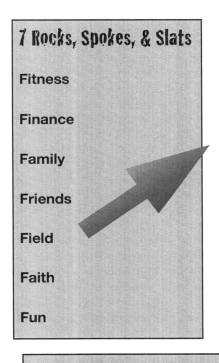

7 Ways to Grow Your Young Living Field

#1- Become your wife's best customer

#2- Read two books about essential oils

#3- Download a podcast

#4- Find someone to tell you a few things

#5- Go and see something

#6- Pick one way to help your wife

#7- Understand the compensation plan

The Weekly Review

#1- File all loose papers

#2- Review the previous week's calendar

#3- Preview the next week's calendar- and, often, the week after that.

#4- Identify the big rocks for the week.

#5- Look at what I delegated to others last week.

#6- Evaluate what I want to read / study this week.

#7- Write it down

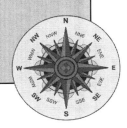

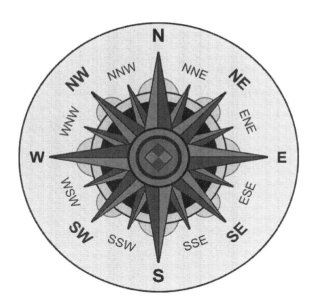

07: Direction: get a little bit better every day

Start walking: Action steps

☐ Answer the following questions related to your "bucket."

> **The main idea:** You don't have to master everything at once. Just improve one thing, and the water level rises for everything else.

• What are your seven slats- or spokes- or rocks?

1. _____

2. _____

3. _____

4. _____

5. _____

6. _____

7. _____

• The two highest slats on my "bucket" are:

   • _____

   • _____

• The two lowest slats are:

   • _____

   • _____

• I can work on my strengths (the highest slats) by (list two specific action steps)- whether it be a class you will attend, a task you will do, a book you will read, a goal you have set, etc.):

   • _____

   • _____

• I can do the following today to raise the lowest:

   • _____

   • _____

• These action steps matter, in terms of where I want to be in the future because…

☐ Write the seven things you will do at your weekly review. You may choose the same seven as I did- or you may choose seven others.

1. _____

2. _____

3. _____

4. _____

5. _____

6. _____

7. _____

☐ Right here, right now **write the day and time that, weekly, you will sit down for at least one hour, on your own, for your own weekly review**[248]:

- Day: _____

- Time: _____

---

[248] As well, I've learned that if I do not schedule the weekly review, it does not happen. And, if I don't have a list of things that I'm going to do during that time, I either a) get stuck doing nothing, or b) get trapped into handling everything in one sitting. Neither option is good. So, I've identified the when (2:00 p.m., right after the little kids go to naps) and the what (my list of seven things I do).

Want to know more?

☐ Read:

    ☐ *Oola*, see Chapter 1, "What is Oola?" and Chapter 2, "Two Roads to Oola."

    ☐ Section Two of the book includes a chapter on each of the seven areas- Fitness (Chapter 3), Finance (Chapter 4), Family (Chapter 5), Field (Chapter 6), Faith (Chapter 7), Friends (Chapter 8), and Fun (Chapter 9).

☐ Listen:

    ☐ To the relevant chapter of the audiobook

☐ Search:

    ☐ Go to www.TheHusbandsFieldGuide.com and download the overview of the comp plan (The Field Guide to the Comp Plan) if you have not already done so. See if the action steps in each chapter help you make next steps in your wife's business.

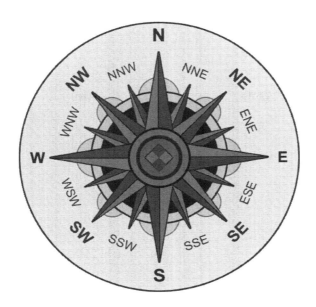

07: The rest is history / Jeremiah's story

I'll never forget the day in 2012, when Monique called me at work. She wanted me to come pick her up from the hospital, where she was working as a nurse at the time. The strange thing was, she was only about half way through her shift.

I remember saying something like," Oh crap, did you get fired?"

Nope, she quit. She had come home crying almost every single day for months and we knew she

Jeremiah McLean is married to Monique, who became a distributor in November 2012. They have two daughters and have been married 15 years.

couldn't keep going this way. But we weren't sure what to do. We had been talking and praying about it for months. Even though I knew this was coming, let me tell you: It was a hard pill to swallow. It was too soon. You see, her paycheck was over half of our income and we were about to close on a new house. But, she'd had enough.

Working in the medical industry, she had become acutely aware of recurring situations that she felt were endangering her patients. She would come home and say things like " We've got to figure out a way to treat ourselves, so we don't have to go to the doctor if we don't have to." We started searching for ways to do that.

Now, at this point we were pretty anti- anything natural, so we really didn't even think about that. Like, we actually made fun of our natural-minded friends (sorry Michael and Anna), just being honest here.

One day we were eating dinner at Les and Kelli's house and they mentioned essential oils. We were like "Yeah, yeah whatever, that's just weird" (at least that's what I was thinking at the time). Then one day Monique and Kelli went out to a mutual friend's farm. Monique had a small allergic reaction to the pollen and stuff and Kelli talked her into trying some lavender. Much to her surprise, it worked! It actually gave her relief right on the spot. Of course, she comes home and tells me about it and I'm like yeah, whatever. Next thing I know she is trying to figure out how to get enough money to buy a starter kit.

Now, I'm thinking here we go again. Something else my wife wants to buy and I'll be paying on for the rest of my life. You know like bead jewelry, some online reading thing for the kids that they never used, scrapbooking, etc. However, one of the many awesome things about my wife is that if she wants something, she will figure out how to make the money to get it. She has a brilliant mind for sales and business, so I wasn't too worried about it.

A few days later the kit comes in the mail. Honestly my first thought was " Is that all I get for $150???"

Then we started using them and Holy Cow they worked! We used them for stomach issues, sleeping and a few other things at first. After doing some research to see what else we could use them for, I realized I could use them for my allergies.

Now, at this point I'm still a pretty big skeptic, it's just my natural inclination to question everything. You can ask anyone that knows me, I never take the easy answer. But I have severe allergies. You know, like have a bottle of meds at work, in my car and at home. So, I was thinking, this is something big we can really put to the test. Then it happened: They actually worked! The years of sneezing, itching, watery eyes were gone with no OTC medicine. I really couldn't believe how well it actually worked! And it only required a few drops a day from that tiny bottle in the starter kit, WOW. I was sold at that point.

Well, the next month Monique discovered the world of "special promos" from Young Living. Of course I'm thinking, here we go, trying to suck me into buying something every month. At that point we were flat broke. We had sold almost everything we owned and moved into a very small house. We were even down to one car. A '98 4runner without AC and the key stuck in the ignition. I'm talking the kind of broke that you question where the next meal is coming from. And Monique wants to know if she can spend $190 to get the "special promo." Is she crazy?!? Again one of the great things about her is that she will find a way.

Andrew

So, I say to her, "Why don't you talk about it on Facebook and see if anyone is interested in getting some?" Then she does something that I think altered the course of our lives forever. She doesn't try to sell anything. She simply posts that she has been using essential oils and lists all the things that they have helped us with. And a funny thing happened. People started blowing up her inbox. They started calling, texting and messaging her like crazy. They were desperate and were willing to try anything to get some relief from their issues. She ended up getting like $1,000 in orders that week!

She had started out saying she didn't want to have anything to do with the business side of this company. In all honesty, we've had quite a few nasty experiences with networking marketing. But this was different. We were just sharing our stories and people were coming out of the woodwork to get it. It was easy and fun. We felt like we were actually helping people instead of selling them something. It was fulfilling. It was at that moment that she started praying, "Lord is this what You want me to do?"

Every January our church does a time of prayer and fasting. So Monique did that. She prayed and fasted for 21 days. She decided that if she was going to do this business, the Lord would have to give her a specific vision for it, because she wasn't going to do it without Him. Trust me, we've tried to do things that way before. Not fun. Even during that time, people kept asking question after question. At the end of the prayer and fasting period, she had a clear direction and vision from the Lord. Shortly thereafter, she started a FB group because she was getting so many questions and getting overwhelmed trying to answer everyone. That group is now called The Lemon Drop Lounge and has 40,000+ members. And the rest is history.

So really this business is about 3 things for us:

1. It's a God thing. He gets all the credit. It wouldn't be anything without Him.

2. We don't sell oils. We just share our story

3. We never push people about doing the business.

It is our hope and prayer that people will come to love them as much as we do and will naturally want to tell their friends, family and sometimes random strangers about them.

— Jeremiah McLean, Monique's husband

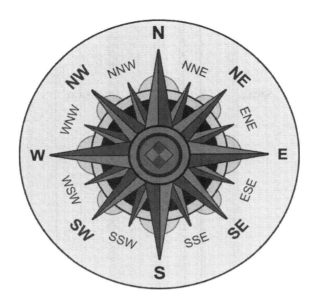

Final thought: keep enjoying the next best step

I found myself getting anxious while we were in Hawaii. Inside, I reasoned to myself something like this:

"Oh, my goodness! We just got into this business. Your wife has been doing this without you and you've lost precious profitable time. You've got to get moving, you've got to start building, you need to get to work! Now!"

> ***Main idea:*** Your future is not going anywhere without you. In fact, it's leisurely waiting for you to arrive. Continue taking the next best step. And enjoy the journey.

Then, the Lord spoke to me and said, "Stop…" A gentle wave of peace flooded me as He continued speaking, "You didn't get here on your own. I brought you here. Me. Not you." Then, "I'll finish it. I'll complete it."

I was reminded of things that I've read in the Bible. Things like:

"...being confident of this, that He who began a good work in you will carry it on to completion..."[249]

And,

"So live in Christ Jesus the Lord in the same way as you received him."[250]

The Lord was clear with me that this entire journey was His idea. He started it. He'll finish it. And, yes, I know the verses are talking about grace and His amazing forgiveness- but they also speak about *all of life and* of how He relates to us now. We don't *just* "enter" into life with Him by grace, grace is how it all continues...

After seeing the incredible opportunity before us, something the Lord totally dropped into our lives when we weren't looking for it, I somehow felt like I. now, had to complete it on my own- and that I had to rush and do it in just a few month's time. Nothing could be more untrue. The One who brought us to the business in His perfect timing will complete it. I have His guarantee that we'll arrive at the perfect destination at just the right time.

You do, too.

As guys, we tend to look at massive goals and try to crush them in an absurdly short amount of time. We go hog-wild and lift weights like a mad man. For a week. We're going

> ... we're back to that "incremental change" thing. Yes, a bunch of little things strung together make a big distance.

to be Mr. Universe or win the Cross-fit championships. We wine and dine our wives like Romeo for the weekend to try and make up for lost time. We're going to be Casanova. We then feel like failures when we falter on accomplishing something that we legitimately tried to do in an unrealistic amount of time.

We forget that the way to eat an elephant remains... you know... one bite at a time. We forget that a marathon is simply 78,600 steps; one right after the other.[251] In other words, we're back to that "incremental change" thing. Yes, a bunch of little things strung together make a big distance.

---

[249] Philippians 1:6, NIV

[250] Colossians 2:6, CEB- Common English Bible

[251] Average runner = 3,000 steps per mile. See http://www.chacha.com/question/how-many-steps-does-the-average-marathon-runner-take-in-a-marathon, accessed 04/16/2014.

One of my favorite Bible passages is Ephesians 2:8-10. Paul writes, "this is not your own doing; it is the gift of God, not a result of works, so that no one may boast. For we are his workmanship, created in Christ Jesus for good works, which **God prepared beforehand, that we should walk in them.**"252 He reminds us of the the same thing the Lord spoke to me that night on the Big Island- "I brought you here. And I've created something for you to walk in… I'll see it through. You enjoy the next steps and don't worry about it."

Because of verses like Paul's, I believe Jesus is *already* in the future. He's in the present, but He's in the future, too. That is, right now, He's walking me- and walking you- incrementally to some great thing He's *already* planned. And even though He's *here* now, He's waiting *there* to celebrate that destination, as well as, every milestone along the way.

Keep walking. Your future is not going anywhere without you. In fact, it's leisurely waiting for you to arrive. Continue taking the next best step. And enjoy the journey.

Grace and peace,

Andrew

---

252 English Standard Version. Emphasis added.

Final thoughts: keep enjoying the next best step

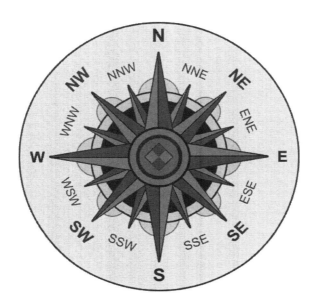

Resources for further study

This resource page includes lists of the following:

- Books referenced in this material
- Documents referenced
- Audio teachings referenced
- Videos referenced
- Websites referenced

Books referenced in this material

Amdahl, Troy and Dave Braun, *Oola*

Covey, Stephen, *The Seven Habits of Highly Effective People*

Brooke, Richard Bliss, *The Four Year Career*

Ferriss, Tim, *The Four-Hour Work Week*

Gladwell, Malcolm, *The Outliers*

Hyatt, Michael, *Life Plan* (e-book)

Johnson, Scott, *Surviving When Modern Medicine Fails*

Life Science Publishing, *Essential Oils Desk Reference*

Life Science Publishing, *Essential Oils Pocket Reference*

Life Science Publishing, *School of Nature's Remedies*

Maxwell, John, *The 21 Irrefutable Laws of Leadership*

Miller, Dan, *48 Days to the Work You Love*

Stanley, Andy, *The Principle of the Path*

Stewart, David, *Healing Oils of the Bible*

Young, D. Gary, *An Introduction to Young Living Essential Oils*

Young, D. Gary, *Aromatherapy: The Essential Beginning*

Documents referenced

"2013 U.S. Income Disclosure Statement" (Young Living)

"Compensation Plan," trifold brochure, item number 4720 (Young Living)

"Young Living Terms and Definitions for the Compensation Plan"

Audio teachings referenced

Andy Stanley's leadership podcast: https://itunes.apple.com/us/podcast/andy-stanley-leadership-podcast/id290055666?mt=2

Our Simple Training: www.OurSimpleTraining.com/Monday-Night-Calls

Young Living's podcast on iTunes: https://itunes.apple.com/us/podcast/young-living-education/id303198270?mt=2

Videos referenced

James and Stacy McDonald's teaching videos:

- "Starting a Young Living Business," 39:22 minutes, located at https://vimeo.com/68374318

- "The Rising Star Bonus!" 6:30 minutes, at https://vimeo.com/71178056

- "The Accidental Paycheck," 6:33 minutes, at https://vimeo.com/74031607

Websites referenced

Halo Aina- Royal Hawaiian Sandalwood (www.HaloAina.com)

The Village (www.WelcomeToTheVillage.net) and The Village Thrift (www.TheVillageThrift.net)

Young Living (www.YoungLiving.com)

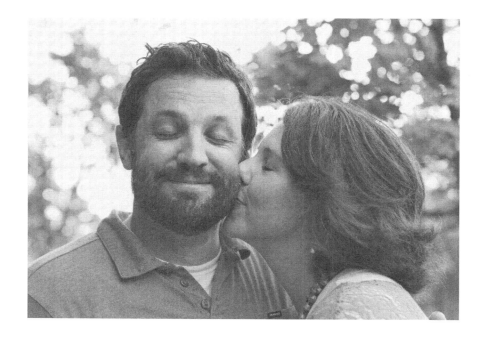

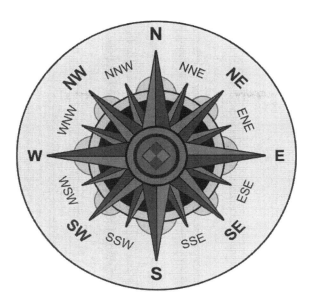

About the author

I'm a thinker, a writer, a teacher... a guy who's led in churches and nonprofits, a guy who's preached and taught and done a bunch of other stuff, too. I've been overwhelmed by my Father's grace.

My fabulous wife loves serving women when they are birthing their babies (*doula* is the word). She teaches about natural childbirth, she home schools our children, and she prays. When she does, she hears the Lord. Less than a year ago, she started a successful home-based essential oil business as a Young Living distributor. I'm way behind on the learning curve, but am honored to be on this journey with her.

We have nine kids. The two most common questions we get are:

- "Are they all yours?" (meaning, ours together- or were some hers and some mine and then we got married. Answer: They are all "ours together"- Seven biological and two are adopted from Uganda. *And*,

- "Have you figured out what causes it?" (or, some version of that, i.e., Do you have a TV?, etc.). Answer: What do you think? Do you think we've figured it out?

The kids are incredible. They pray, they serve, they love doing ministry. And, of course (since they're kids), they love swashbuckling, too. FYI, they always get a prize when they're in public and someone remarks about how well behaved they are, so throw them a bone next time you see them. They'll never forget you. *I promise.*

Our kids' ages range from 13 down to 1. Besides these, another precious one is in heaven.

They're quite diverse: A budding author who likes to sing and dance (and is currently working on a kids version of this book). A tender young lady who is nurturing, kind and an amazing gymnast. She's also known as our faith healer (no kidding). A young boy who loves to preach, has mastered Legos, and has set up his own vending machine business. Another young boy who is tender and compassionate- and will drop whatever he's doing to help you. A young boy who is genuine, smiles constantly and loves people- and people love him. Another boy who is larger than life and can out-dance anyone. Period. The Sweet (self-explanatory, especially after you meet him and listen to his buttery

voice). The youngest girl, we affectionately call "Mini"- not to be confused with her determination and perseverance, though. The baby, who's just happy to be around and share his opinion at will. He is full of life and happiness and joy. Yep, that's 6 boys and 3 girls!

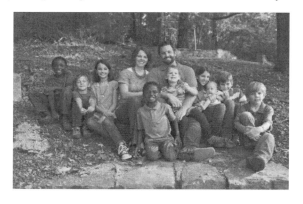

Most of what we do, we do together. You'll see us (together) doing various service projects around our city, riding bikes at the park, hiking at Ruffner Mountain, staying up 'til midnight for a "movie night" (the kids' favorite- the way they count in all birthdays, holidays, and anything else you can think of), or going on some other adventure.

So, that's my highlight reel. Thanks for your interest in the book. If you have questions, comments, or just want to connect, you can find me online at www.TheHusbandsFieldGuide.com, or via email: AndrewEJenkins@aol.com. And, yes, I'm on FaceBook and Twitter and everything else!

Made in the USA
San Bernardino, CA
06 June 2014